MediSoft Made Easy

MediSoft Made Easy
A Step-by-Step Approach

Lillian D. Burke, AAS, BBA, MA
Middlesex County College

Barbara Weill, BA, MA, PhD, AA
Middlesex County College

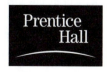

Upper Saddle River, New Jersey 07458

Library of Congress Cataloging-in-Publication Data

Burke, Lillian.
    Medisoft made easy : a step-by-step approach / Lillian D. Burke,
Barbara Weill.
        p. cm.
    Includes bibliographical references and index.
    ISBN 0-13-097710-1
    1. Medisoft.   2. Medical informatics.   3. Medical
offices—Automation.   I. Weill, Barbara.   II. Title.
    R858 .B856 2003
    651′.961′0285—dc21
                                                    2002155151

Notice: The authors and the publisher of this volume have taken care that the information and technical recommendations contained herein are based on research and expert consultation, and are accurate and compatible with the standards generally accepted at the time of publication. Nevertheless, as new information becomes available, changes in clinical and technical practices become necessary. The reader is advised to carefully consult manufacturers' instructions and information material for all supplies and equipment before use, and to consult with a healthcare professional as necessary. This advice is especially important when using new supplies or equipment for clinical purposes. The authors and publisher disclaim all responsibility for any liability, loss, injury, or damage incurred as a consequence, directly or indirectly, of the use and application of any of the contents of this volume.

Publisher: Julie Levin Alexander
Assistant to Publisher: Regina Bruno
Senior Acquisitions Editor: Mark Cohen
Assistant Editor: Melissa Kerian
Editorial Assistant: Mary Ellen Ruitenberg
Senior Marketing Manager: Nicole Benson
Marketing Assistant: Janet Ryerson
Product Information Manager: Rachele Strober
Director of Manufacturing and Production: Bruce Johnson
Production Managing Editor: Patrick Walsh
Production Liaison: Alex Ivchenko

Production Editor: Karen Berry
Manufacturing Manager: Ilene Sanford
Manufacturing Buyer: Pat Brown
Design Director: Cheryl Asherman
Senior Design Coordinator: Maria Guglielmo Walsh
Cover Designer: Christopher Weigand
Manager of Media Production: Amy Peltier
New Media Project Manager: Lisa Rinaldi
Composition: Pine Tree Composition, Inc.
Printing & Binding: Courier Westford
Cover Printer: Phoenix Color

MediSoft is a registered trademark of NDC Health.

Pearson Education Ltd., *London*
Pearson Education Australia PTY, Limited, *Sydney*
Pearson Education Singapore, Pte. Ltd.
Pearson Education North Asia Ltd., *Hong Kong*
Pearson Education Canada, Ltd., *Toronto*
Pearson Education de Mexico, S.A. de C.V.
Pearson Education—Japan, Tokyo
Pearson Education Malaysia, Pte. Ltd

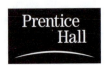

10 9 8 7 6 5 4 3 2 1
ISBN 0-13-097710-1

Contents

Preface

Computer technology is transforming all aspects of our lives, including how we think, analyze, educate, buy, protect, and care for one another. The term *medical informatics* refers to the use of computer technology in health care and its delivery. The skillful use of computers and software programs is the key to success in virtually all of today's professions. This is particularly true in health care fields, where students, health care providers, and office personnel need to use computer technology. *MediSoft Made Easy* addresses the medical office worker and student of medical office administration. MediSoft is computer software that can help computerize administrative functions in the medical office, including entering and editing patient information, provider information, and case information; entering and editing transaction charges, payments, and adjustment information; creating and managing claims; and creating and printing various kinds of reports. All this information is saved in tables in a relational database (an organized collection of related data).

The first chapter of *MediSoft Made Easy* is a general introduction to medical informatics. Chapter 2 familiarizes the reader with the Windows environment and basic Windows terminology. Chapter 3 is an overview of using MediSoft in the medical office. It should be noted that this book is written for a student in a classroom setting. Therefore, some of the events take place in an unrealistic time frame; for example, in Chapter 10, the discussion assumes the insurer pays a claim the same day a patient is seen. This would never happen.

Chapters 4–11 are a step-by-step hands-on introduction to MediSoft. We approached MediSoft as novice users would approach it, and present it to the student in the same fashion. We begin with an overview of MediSoft; and proceed to introduce each part of the program. In Chapter 4, the reader learns how to make appointments using MediSoft's scheduling software, the Appointment Book. In Chapter 5, the reader learns how to enter patient and case information. Chapters 6 and 7 introduce the reader to entering transactions and processing claims. In Chapters 8 and 9, the reader learns how to print and design reports. In Chapter 10, we review all the previous tasks by taking the student through the process of creating a new database for a new practice. Some tasks, such as using MediSoft utilities, cannot be performed in a classroom setting. However, these aspects of the program are surveyed in Chapter 11 so that the student has at least some familiarity with them in a real working environment.

An Appendix is recommended for students who have no knowledge of computers. It introduces the student to computers and computer literacy, including basic computer terminology.

We would like to thank the following people for reviewing this book in manuscript form: Sharon L. Charlton, RN, CMA, Medical Assisting Program Director, Lee County High Tech Center Central, Fort Myers, Florida; George W. Fakhoury, MD, Medical Director, Medical Assisting Program, Silicon Valley College, Concord, California; Lisa Nagle, CMA, Bsed, Medical Assisting Program Director, Augusta Technical College, Augusta, Georgia; Jean M. Runyon, Professor, Technical Studies Department and Faculty Development Coordinator, College of Southern Maryland, La Plata, Maryland; Terry Young, MS, Medical Careers Program Director, Latter Day Saints Business College, Salt Lake City, Utah; and Deena Nathan-Strauss, President, QHB, Inc., Boca Raton, Florida.

Lillian D. Burke
Barbara Weill

MediSoft Made Easy

An Introduction to Medical Informatics

Chapter Outline

- Learning Objectives
- Medical Informatics
- Administrative Applications of Computer Technology in the Medical Office Using MediSoft
- Clinical Applications
- Special-Purpose Applications
- Telemedicine
- Privacy and Security of Medical Information
- Health Insurance Portability and Accountability Act of 1996 (HIPAA)
- Chapter Summary
- Key Words
- Review Exercises

Learning Objectives

Upon completion of this chapter, the reader will be able to

- Define medical informatics
- Define clinical, special-purpose, and administrative applications of computer technology in health care and its delivery
- Define telemedicine
- Define administrative applications of computer technology in health care, with specific reference to MediSoft
- Discuss issues related to the privacy and security of medical information
- Be aware of the privacy protections of the Health Insurance Portability and Accountability Act (HIPAA)

MEDICAL INFORMATICS

The use of computers and computer information technology in health care and its delivery is called **medical informatics**. Traditionally, the application of computer technology in health care is divided into three categories. The **clinical** uses of computers include anything that has to do with direct patient care, including diagnosis, treatment, and monitoring. **Special-purpose applications** include the use of computers in teaching and some aspects of pharmacy. **Administrative** applications include office management, scheduling, and billing tasks. MediSoft and other programs like it are specifically designed for medical office management. **Telemedicine**—the delivery of health care over telecommunications lines—crosses all traditional boundaries and includes clinical, special-purpose, and administrative applications.

Beginning with the computerization of hospital administrative tasks in the 1960s, the role of digital technology in medical care and its delivery has expanded at an ever-increasing pace. Today, computers play a part in every aspect of health care.

ADMINISTRATIVE APPLICATIONS OF COMPUTER TECHNOLOGY IN THE MEDICAL OFFICE USING MEDISOFT

As you recall, administrative applications include office management tasks, scheduling, and billing. These are tasks that need to be performed in any office. However, some of these activities are slightly different in a health care environment, so programs are needed that take into account the special needs of a medical office.

MediSoft is a program specifically designed to computerize basic administrative functions in a health care environment. It allows the user to organize information by patient, by case, and by provider. It enables the user to schedule patient appointments with a computer; take electronic progress notes; create lists of codes for diagnosis, treatment, and insurance; submit claims to primary, secondary, and tertiary insurers; and receive payment electronically. MediSoft is appropriate to the **bucket billing**, or **balance billing**, that medical offices must use to accommodate two or three insurers, who must be billed in a timely fashion *before* the patient is billed. Moreover, because MediSoft is a **relational database** (an organized collection of related data), information input in one part of the program can be linked to information in another part of the program. Billing information and financial status are easily available in MediSoft. Tables can be searched for any information, and this information can be presented in finished form in one of the many report designs provided, including various kinds of billing reports. If no report design meets the user's need, a customized report can easily be designed and generated by the user.

CLINICAL APPLICATIONS

In hospitals, nurses and staff can oversee patient care from centrally located cameras and monitoring stations that provide instant access to a patient's condition. For help with diagnosis, sophisticated digital imaging techniques, including **Computerized Tomography (CT scans)**, **Magnetic Resonance Imaging (MRIs)**, and **Positron Emission Tomography (PET scans)**, are supplementing the use of X rays, as digital images replace images on film. **Expert systems**, which turn the computer into an expert in one specific area, can help medical personnel diagnose and treat conditions they have never seen. There are many expert systems in medicine: POEMS, for example, deals specifically with postoperative complications. INTERNIST is an expert on bacterial infections. Robotic devices take part in surgeries. ROBODOC drills the hole in the femur for cementless hip replacements. AESOP holds the endoscope in laparoscopic surgeries. DaVinci has performed long-distance surgeries; for example, a patient in Bosnia was operated on by a robot controlled by a doctor in Germany.

The microprocessor, a computer on a chip of silicon, which is embedded in many home appliances, is also embedded in many medical appliances. It is used to control heart pacemakers. Microprocessors control other medical devices also, from defibrillators, to IV (intravenous) pumps, to incubators. What makes a microprocessor-controlled device unique is that, like larger computers, it can be programmed, and it can respond to changing conditions. The microprocessor is also found in electronic prostheses (replacement limbs and organs). This has made possible prosthetic limbs that can receive the electrical signal from the residual limb and move, for example, fingers that move independently of each other and play the piano; feet that walk and run; and hands that feel hot and cold. Computerized functional electrical stimulation (CFES) applied to the outside of a paralyzed limb can simulate a workout and can even return movement to some paralyzed limbs.

SPECIAL-PURPOSE APPLICATIONS

Computers have made a major, positive contribution to the pharmaceutical industry. Computers can be used in every facet of pharmacy, from helping design medications to warning of possible adverse drug events, to filling prescriptions and delivering medication. Computers may help in the design of new medications. Rational drug design is based on the assumption that the body is a collection of molecules; when one molecule causes harm, it is necessary to find another molecule to bind to it and correct it. The correcting molecule must fit it like a key to a lock. Numerous calculations are necessary, and then a model of the molecule can be built. Before computers, the calculations had to be performed by hand and the model built of wire. This might take years. Now a powerful computer does the calculations in a fraction of the time and simulates the molecule on a computer screen. Computers can also help design drugs by scanning databases of compounds and trying any one likely to work—a computer's process of trial and error. Computers made possible the **Human Genome Project**, which sought to understand the genetic makeup of a human being. Part of the Human Genome Project attempted to gain an understanding of the genetic bases of diseases. This understanding could lead to the development of medications.

The use of computers in health care education is also considered a special-purpose use. Programs such as **ADAM** and **ILIAD** have been used for years: ADAM is used to help teach anatomy, and ILIAD teaches clinical problem-solving skills. Today simulations are used to help teach skills in dentistry, surgery, and nursing.

Huge databases of medical information on the Internet have made it possible for anyone with an Internet connection to find medical information and misinformation. This may radically change the visit to the doctor. The patient may have more up-to-date knowledge of a particular treatment or condition than the doctor. Much of the information on the Internet is incorrect, and we recommend reputable sites like the University of Iowa or the government-maintained **MEDLARS** databases. The largest of these is **MEDLINE**, which includes abstracts of articles from around the world and is searchable by using PubMed (MEDLINE's search engine). However reliable the site, do NOT substitute Internet information for a visit to a health care provider.

TELEMEDICINE

Connectivity and **networking** have made the field of telemedicine possible. Telemedicine involves the delivery of health care over telecommunications lines. It includes everything from the sharing of radiological images over a network (the oldest form of telemedicine), to distance exams via videoconferencing, to telepsychiatry, teledermatology, teleoncology, and even distance surgery. Via a telemedical hookup, visiting nurses in New Jersey see some patients without leaving the office. A computer named HANC (Home-Assisted Nursing Care) allows a nurse to take blood pressure and listen to a patient's heart without visiting the patient. HANC also reminds the patient to take his or her medicine, yelling louder and louder until the patient responds, and finally if there is no response, notifying a nurse. Telemedicine delivers health care in some prisons. It is also used in problem pregnancies to get an expert consult without a patient having to wait weeks for an appointment or travel what may be long distances. In addition, telemedicine has been used to deliver psychiatric services to hearing impaired clients and to deliver health services to a homeless shelter. There have been no comprehensive studies comparing telemedicine and conventional medicine. Early indications are, however, that telemedicine compares favorably with conventional medicine.

PRIVACY AND SECURITY OF MEDICAL INFORMATION

Computers have made significant contributions to health care and its delivery. But not all of the contributions of computers are positive. Computers and networks endanger the **privacy** of personal information. Information is kept in databases and on computer networks on many aspects of our lives: the phone calls we make, property we own, the Web sites we visit, credit card purchases we make, our marital status and the number and ages of our children, our medical records, and our credit status. Much of this information was always gathered. However, it usually was filed away in small courthouses (marriage licenses, property ownership). It was scattered physically and difficult to find. Now, much of this information is kept on computer networks, including the Internet. The Medical Information Bureau, an organization made up of insurance companies, keeps the medical records of anyone with insurance. Until April 14, 2003, this information can be shared with other insurance companies and with employers. It can be used by employers to deny employment or promotions. In April 2003, new regulations regarding the privacy of medical information go into effect under the Health Insurance Portability and Accountability Act of 1996 (HIPAA).

The paper medical record is currently being replaced by the **electronic medical record (EMR)**.* The EMR may be stored in a hospital's private network, but it may also be kept on the Internet.

*For a complete discussion of medical privacy issues, see Lillian Burke and Barbara Weill, *Information Technology for the Health Professions* (Upper Saddle River, NJ: Prentice Hall, 2000), Chapter 4.

There are many benefits to the EMR: Because your record is available anywhere there is a computer on the network, the EMR helps guarantee continuity of care; each of your health care providers knows your full medical history and can therefore provide better care. If you are in an accident in New Jersey, for example, but live in California, your record is a mouse-click away. The EMR is legible and complete. Despite its benefits, the EMR raises serious privacy issues. Any network can be broken into, and your medical information can be stolen and misused. A great deal of medical information is private. No one wants their psychiatric diagnosis, HIV status, or children's head lice broadcast to the neighborhood. Privacy issues are also raised by telemedicine, which transmits medical information across state lines via telecommunications lines. The states have traditionally provided protection for medical information; however, once the information crosses state lines, it does not have state legal protection.

Are there ways of protecting sensitive information or guaranteeing **security**? There are various attempts to guarantee that only people authorized to see the information can access it. Computers can be kept in a locked room and authorized personnel can be issued keys or swipe cards; **PIN numbers (personal identification numbers)** and **passwords** can be used to identify authorized users; or **biometric methods** can be used—handprints or fingerprints, face scans, body scans, iris scans. **Firewalls** (electronic blocks) are used to keep people out of private networks. **Callback systems** are used to attempt to protect networks. A user calls in; the network hangs up and calls the user back at an authorized phone. None of these methods is foolproof. Keys and cards can be lost or stolen; PINs and passwords can be forgotten or shared. **Encryption** (scrambling) of sensitive data, so that only authorized personnel have the **decryption** software, is also being implemented.

Restricting access to computer systems to people who are authorized is not really enough, because the FBI estimates that people who have legitimate access commit more than half of all computer crimes. With our current fragmented health care system, more and more people are authorized to see a medical record. **HMOs (health maintenance organizations)** are replacing traditional practice. In one hospital stay, think of how many people share your record—from clerks in a pharmacy, to kitchen personnel in the hospital kitchen, to technicians, nurses, and doctors. Many of these people are not trained in medical ethics, and have little interest in protecting a patient's privacy. Of course, it would help to train all hospital personnel in medical ethics, to train them not to share information, and to use a password-protected screensaver. However, this would not solve the problem. When a person gets medical insurance, he or she signs away all privacy rights. Until these privacy and security problems are solved, the EMR will not fulfill its promise to make complete and accurate medical information available to those who need it.

THE HEALTH INSURANCE PORTABILITY AND ACCOUNTABILITY ACT (HIPAA)

In 1996, Congress passed the **Health Insurance Portability and Accountability Act (HIPAA)**. The law "encourag[ed] electronic transactions, but it also required new safeguards to protect the security and confidentiality" of health information (HHS Fact Sheet, http://ssps.hhs.gov/admissimp/final/profact2.htm [March 9, 2001; January 10, 2002]). The new safeguards do not override stronger state protections. However, HIPAA will provide national minimum privacy protections in April 2003.

Under HIPAA, if Congress failed to pass patient privacy protection, the Department of Health and Human Services (HHS) was required to issue regulations. HHS issued proposed regulations in November 1999, and the regulations went into effect on April 14, 2001; health plans, clearinghouses, and providers who use electronic billing and funds transfer have until April 14, 2003, to comply. The new regulations cover "[a]ll medical records and other individually identifiable health information used or disclosed by a covered entity in any form, whether electronically, on paper, or orally." Higher standards apply to psychotherapy notes, which are not considered part of a medical record under this law, and "are never intended to be shared with anyone else." The law applies to both public and private providers and institutions. Providers must give patients a written explanation of how their health information may be used; patients may see, copy, and request changes in their medical records. Providers need a patient's consent before using his or her information. Health information may no longer be used by employers or banks to make decisions regarding employment or loans. Except for the sharing of information for the purpose of treatment, "disclosures . . . will be limited to the minimum necessary" (HHS Fact Sheet, http://ssps.hhs.gov/admissimp/final/profact2.htm [March 9, 2001; January 10, 2002]).

Health care providers and institutions may design their own procedures to meet the new standards; however, they must be written and must include the following information: who has access to patient information, how this information will be used, and the conditions under which it may be shared. Health care providers are responsible for seeing that those with whom they do business also protect patient privacy. Employees must be trained to respect patient privacy and follow privacy procedures, and one person must be chosen to ensure that the privacy procedures are followed. Under specific conditions, health information may be shared without the patient's consent (e.g., for public health needs, research, and some law enforcement activities, and when the interests of national defense and security are involved). Under HIPAA, violations of the law can be punished by both civil and criminal penalties (HHS Fact Sheet, http:// ssps.hhs.gov/admissimp/final/profact2.htm [March 9, 2001; January 10, 2002]).

The projected cost of implementation of the HIPAA regulations is $17.6 billion over ten years. However, it is also projected that implementing electronic billing and electronic funds transfer will save $29.9 billion (HHS Fact Sheet, http://ssps.hhs.gov/admissimp/ final/profact2.htm [March 9, 2001; January 10, 2002]).

Chapter Summary

- Computers are used throughout our society, including in health care and its delivery.
- The use of computers in health care and its delivery is called medical informatics.
- Administrative applications include the use of computers in a medical office. MediSoft allows the user to computerize medical office management functions.
- Clinical applications use computers in direct patient care such as diagnosis, monitoring, and treatment.
- Special-purpose applications include drug design and educational uses.
- Telemedicine is the delivery of health care over telecommunications lines, and includes administrative, clinical, and special-purpose applications.
- Medical information is available on-line in electronic form. The electronic medical record (EMR) provides continuity of care. The privacy and security issues surrounding the EMR must be addressed. Some attempts at restricting access to medical records include training personnel, PINs and passwords for authorized personnel, encryption, firewalls, and callback systems. Further steps must be taken to guarantee the security of medical information.
- The Health Insurance Portability and Accountability Act (HIPAA) encourages the use of the electronic medical record, and provides minimum national standards for the protection of medical information.

Key Words

ADAM
Administrative application
Balance billing
Biometric
Bucket billing
Callback systems
Clinical application
Computerized Tomography (CT
    Scans)
Connectivity
Decryption
Electronic medical record
    (EMR)
Encryption
Expert systems
Firewall
Health Insurance Portability and
    Accountability Act (HIPAA)
HMO (health maintenance
    organization)

Human Genome Project
ILIAD
Magnetic Resonance Imaging
    (MRIs)
Medical informatics
MediSoft
MEDLARS
MEDLINE
Networking
Password
PIN number (personal identifi-
    cation number)
Positron Emission Tomography
    (PET) Scan
Privacy
Relational database
Security
Special-purpose application
Telemedicine

REVIEW EXERCISES

Define the following terms:

Medical Informatics

Administrative Applications

Telemedicine

Clinical Applications

Special-Purpose Applications

Briefly discuss the following:

1. Discuss the positive and negative contributions of the electronic medical record.
2. Discuss the privacy problems associated with telemedicine.
3. The Health Insurance Portability and Accountability Act (HIPAA) requires medical offices to design privacy policies. What kind of safeguards would you introduce to protect the privacy of information?

2

A Brief Introduction to the Windows Environment

Chapter Outline

- Introduction
- Windows 2000
  - Parts of a Window
  - Parts of a Dialog Box
- Chapter Summary
- Key Words
- Review Exercises

Learning Objectives

Upon completing this chapter:

- You will be familiar with the Windows environment and its terminology
- You will be able to describe the parts of a window and a dialog box

INTRODUCTION

This chapter introduces the student to basic Windows vocabulary and concepts. MediSoft for Windows operates in a **Windows** environment. It is necessary to be familiar with Windows terminology to fully appreciate MediSoft.

WINDOWS 2000

Computer hardware cannot function without instructions. These step-by-step instructions are called **programs** or **software**. There are two basic kinds of software: application and system. **Application software** helps to do a specific task; for example, a word processing program helps you type a letter or memo; MediSoft helps computerize administrative functions in a health care environment. **System software** takes care of tasks for the computer. The most important piece of system software is the **operating system (OS)**. Every computer has an operating system that takes care of routine tasks. The operating system is a group of programs that provides a user interface, defining how the user communicates with the computer's hardware. The operating system also coordinates and controls basic input and output, receiving commands from the keyboard, displaying information on the screen. It also organizes and tracks your files in memory and on disk. The operating system must be loaded in the computer's memory for the computer to do anything. Loading the operating system is called **booting**.

Today most personal computers use Windows as an operating system. Windows allows the user to communicate with the computer through a **graphical user interface** (GUI) by using a **mouse** and clicking on **icons** (pictures and symbols).

A mouse is an input device attached to the computer by a cable. It has one, two, or three buttons on the top and a ball on the bottom. When you move the mouse across a flat surface (a mouse pad), a mouse pointer moves on the screen.

The mouse pointer takes on different shapes:

- It is an **arrow** ↗ when selecting or choosing
- An **I-beam** I for editing
- An **hourglass** ⧗ when Windows needs time to process a command
- A **two-headed arrow** ↔ when changing the size of a window
- A **hand** 🖑 to choose help topics.

There are several basic mouse operations:

- **Pointing** is moving the mouse across a flat surface.
- **Clicking** is pressing and releasing the left mouse button.
- **Double-clicking** is quickly pressing and releasing the left mouse button twice.
- **Right-clicking** is clicking the right mouse button. It opens a shortcut menu.
- **Dragging** is holding down the left mouse button while moving the mouse.

Your work area, the screen on which icons and windows are arranged, is called the **desktop**. Across the bottom of the desktop is a **taskbar**. The taskbar displays a button for each open application. At the left of the taskbar is a **Start button**. Clicking Start causes a **menu** (list of choices) to pop up. You can execute most tasks by sliding the mouse pointer to the option you want and clicking. If an option has a left pointing arrowhead next to it, another menu will drop down; move the mouse pointer to that menu, slide it to your selection, and click.

When you first launch Windows, there are several icons on the desktop. An icon is a little picture representing a program or piece of hardware. To open an icon into a window (a rectangular area surrounded by a border), point to the icon and double-click. In Windows, applications (programs) run in windows and documents open in windows.

The Windows Desktop

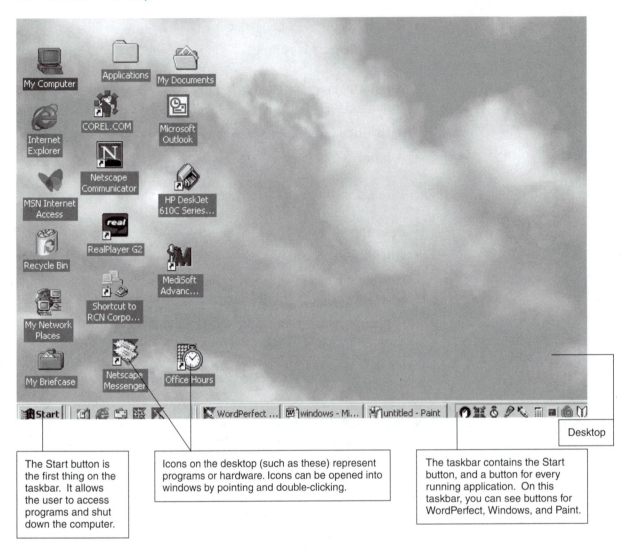

Desktop

The Start button is the first thing on the taskbar. It allows the user to access programs and shut down the computer.

Icons on the desktop (such as these) represent programs or hardware. Icons can be opened into windows by pointing and double-clicking.

The taskbar contains the Start button, and a button for every running application. On this taskbar, you can see buttons for WordPerfect, Windows, and Paint.

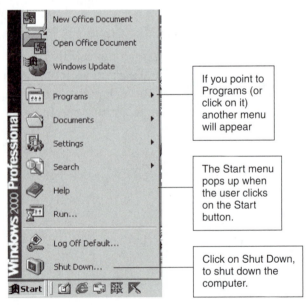

If you point to Programs (or click on it) another menu will appear

The Start menu pops up when the user clicks on the Start button.

Click on Shut Down, to shut down the computer.

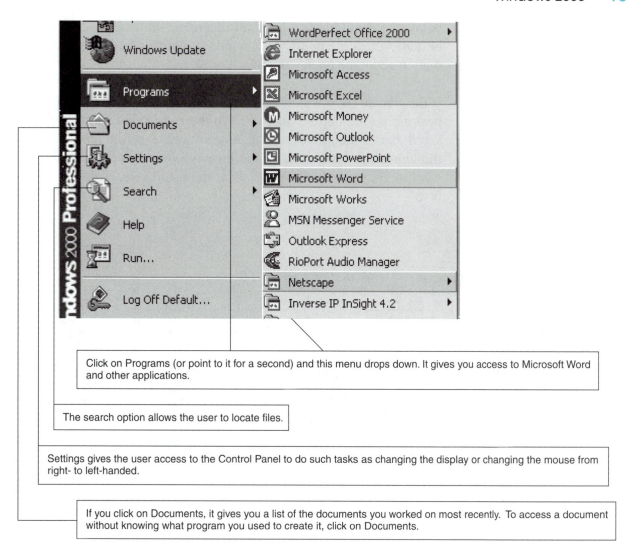

Click on Programs (or point to it for a second) and this menu drops down. It gives you access to Microsoft Word and other applications.

The search option allows the user to locate files.

Settings gives the user access to the Control Panel to do such tasks as changing the display or changing the mouse from right- to left-handed.

If you click on Documents, it gives you a list of the documents you worked on most recently. To access a document without knowing what program you used to create it, click on Documents.

The Parts of a Window

One of the features of the Windows environment is a **common user interface**; this means that every window has similar parts. Across the top is a **title bar** with the **window title** in it. At the right of the title bar are three buttons: the **minimize, maximize** or **restore**, and **close buttons**. Clicking the minimize button does not cause the application to stop running; the button still appears on the taskbar, although you no longer see an open window. Clicking the maximize button causes the window to expand to fill the screen and a restore button to replace the maximize button. Clicking the restore button causes the window to resume its former size. Clicking the close button closes the window; the application is no longer running, and its button is no longer on the taskbar.

Some windows have other components. Below the title bar (in windows that run applications) is a **menu bar**. **Toolbars** may appear below the menu bar and let you execute a command by clicking on a button. Across the bottom of a window, a **status bar** gives you information about the open window.

If the contents of a window are not completely visible, **scroll bars** appear across the bottom and/or down the right side of the window. A scroll bar contains two scroll arrows and a scroll box. To move through a window, click on the arrow pointing in the direction you want to go, or click above or below the scroll box, or drag the scroll box.

The Parts of a Window

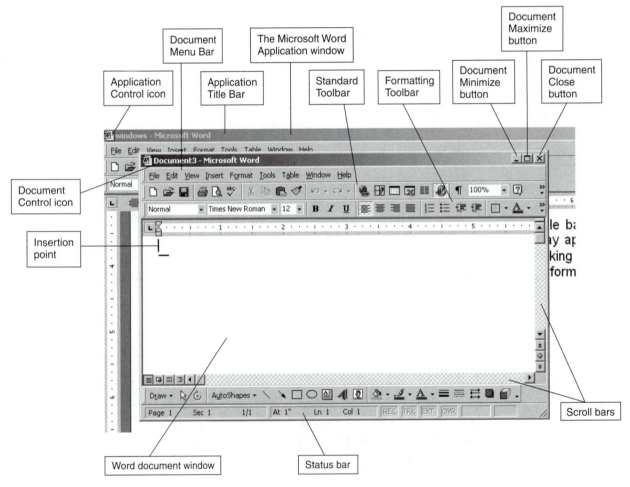

A menu is a list of commands. You display the commands on a menu by pointing to the menu title and clicking or pressing ALT while tapping the underlined letter in the menu name (e.g., ALT-F pulls down the File menu). You can choose a command by clicking on it or typing the underlined letter. When you choose a command that is followed by an ellipsis (three dots . . .), the command is not immediately executed. Instead, a window called a **dialog box** opens. A dialog box is a window used when the computer needs more information. Dialog boxes may have one or more of the following elements:

- **Tabs** look like file folder tabs. They appear at the top of the dialog box and are used to switch to a different page of the dialog box.

- **Text boxes** allow you to enter data.

- **List boxes** display a list of choices. Click on the option to make a choice.

- **Drop-down list boxes** contain a down arrow; click on the arrow to display the choices. Click on the option to make a choice.

- **Command buttons** are rectangular buttons that execute commands. OK and Cancel are common.

- **Check boxes** are square boxes that you can click on or off. More than one may be chosen.

- **Option buttons** are round. Only one may be selected; however, one MUST be selected.

- **Spin boxes** allow you to make a choice by clicking on an up or down arrow.

- **Slide boxes** let you to make a choice by moving a slider bar.

The Parts of a Dialog Box

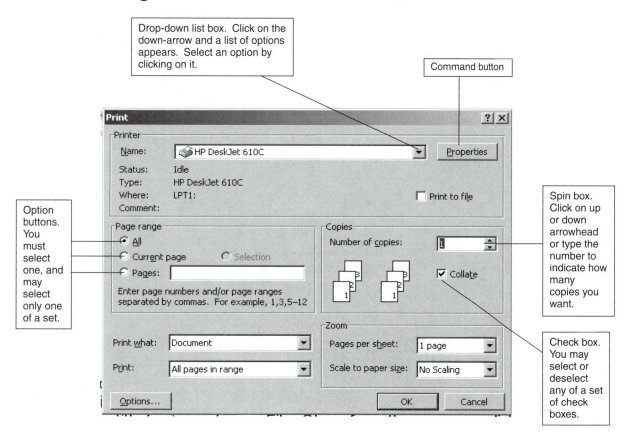

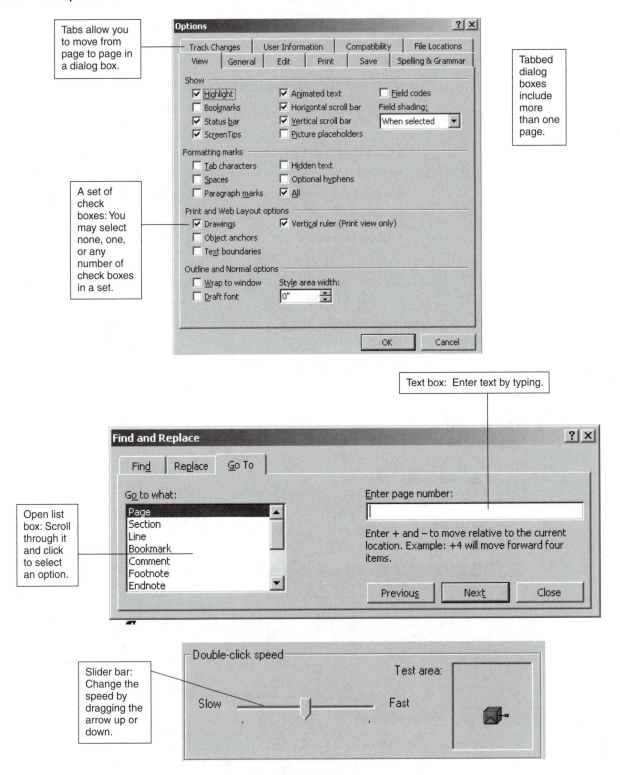

Tabs allow you to move from page to page in a dialog box.

Tabbed dialog boxes include more than one page.

A set of check boxes: You may select none, one, or any number of check boxes in a set.

Text box: Enter text by typing.

Open list box: Scroll through it and click to select an option.

Slider bar: Change the speed by dragging the arrow up or down.

Chapter Summary

- The operating system is a piece of system software that defines the general working environment of a computer. Therefore, it is necessary for the user to be familiar with the operating system.

Application software helps you do a specific task. MediSoft is an application program that helps computerize functions in a medical office environment. The following chapters will introduce the user to MediSoft in a Windows environment.

Key Words

Application software
Arrow
Booting
Check boxes
Clicking
Close button
Command buttons
Common user interface
Desktop
Dialog box
Double-clicking
Dragging
Drop-down list boxes
Formatting toolbar
Graphical user interface (GUI)
Hand
Hourglass
I-beam
Icons
List box
Maximize button
Menu
Menu Bar
Minimize button

Mouse
Option buttons
Operating system
Pointing
Program
Restore button
Right-clicking
Scroll bars
Slide boxes
Software
Spin boxes
Standard toolbar
Start button
Status bar
System software
Tabs
Taskbar
Text boxes
Title bar
Toolbar
Two-headed arrow
Window
Window title
Windows

REVIEW EXERCISES

Fill-in Questions

1. A window called a _____ is used to collect more information for the computer.

2. The user must make _____ choices from a group of option buttons.

3. _____ appear across the top of a many-paged dialog box.

4. A user may choose one or two or three (or none) from a group of _____ boxes.

5. Windows provides a _____ user interface. The user uses a mouse to click on icons.

True/False Questions

1. Windows is an example of system software called an operating system. T/F

2. Booting refers to loading any program into memory. T/F

3. The user is required to make one choice from a set of option buttons. T/F

4. The user must make one choice from a set of four check boxes. T/F

Matching Questions

Match the letter with the correct name:

_____ Formatting toolbar   _____ Ruler

_____ Drop-down list boxes   _____ Minimize button

_____ Menu bar   _____ Standard toolbar

_____ Close button   _____ Maximize button

_____ Title bar

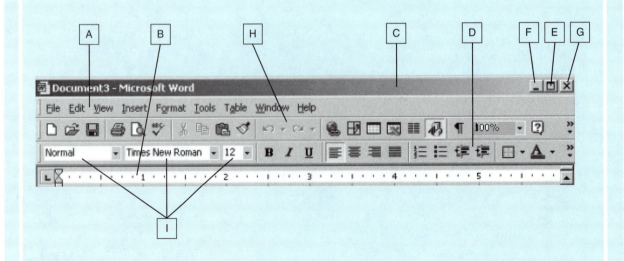

3

An Overview: Using MediSoft in the Medical Office

Chapter Outline

- Learning Objectives
- Introduction
- Database Concepts
- An Overview of MediSoft
  - The Patient Information Form
  - Coding Systems: DRG, ICD, CPT
  - The Electronic Medical Record (EMR)
  - Accounting, Using MediSoft
  - Insurance
  - Claims
  - Accounting Reports
- Chapter Summary
- Key Words
- Review Exercises

Learning Objectives

After completing this chapter, the student will

- Be able to define basic database concepts, including file, table, record, field, and relational database
- Understand the flow of work in a medical office from the patient information form to the electronic medical record, to the submission of insurance claims
- Be able to define the coding systems (DRG, ICD, CPT) and understand their uses
- Describe the role of MediSoft in the accounting process

- Comprehend the differences between types of insurance (fee-for-service, health maintenance organizations, capitated plans, participating provider organizations, etc.)
- Understand the process of claims submission
- Be aware of MediSoft's various accounting reports

INTRODUCTION

MediSoft software can be used by medical administrators and office workers, doctors and other health care workers, and students. It can ease the tasks of administering a practice using a computer. The amount of data and information a modern practice has to collect and organize is overwhelming. MediSoft allows the user to computerize tasks performed every day in any medical environment. All the disparate tasks and pieces of data and information need to be well organized, accessible, and easily linked. Because MediSoft is a relational database, the user can quickly and easily organize, access, and link information from one part of the program to information in any other part of the program.

DATABASE CONCEPTS

A **database** is an organized collection of information. **Database management software (DBMS)** allows the user to enter, organize, and store huge amounts of data and information. The information can then be updated, sorted, resorted, and retrieved. In order to use database management software efficiently, the user should be familiar with certain concepts and definitions. A database **file** holds all related information on an entity, for example, a medical practice. Within each file, there can be several **tables**. Each table holds related information; for example, one table might hold information on a practice's doctors; another holds information on its patients; another on its insurance carriers. A table is made up of related **records**; each record holds all the information on one item in a table. Each patient has a record in the practice's patient table. All the information on one patient makes up that patient's record. Each record is made up of related **fields**. One field holds one piece of information, such as a patient's last name, or Social Security number (SSN), or chart number. One field—the **key field**—uniquely identifies each record in a table. The information in that field cannot be duplicated. The Social Security number is a common key field because no two people have the same SSN. The chart number uniquely identifies each patient's chart. In a relational database such as MediSoft, related tables are linked by sharing a common field.

AN OVERVIEW OF MEDISOFT

MediSoft allows the user to create one database file for each practice. Within each database, information is organized in tables. The tables are linked by sharing a common field.

The Patient Information Form

When a patient schedules an appointment, it is recorded in Medi-Soft's Electronic Appointment Book. At or before a patient's first visit, he or she fills out a Patient Information Form. It includes such personal data as name, address, home and work phones, date of birth, Social Security number, and student status. The patient is also asked to fill in information about his or her spouse or partner.

Medical information is required: allergies, medical history, and current medications. The patient is also asked for the reason for the visit, such as accident or illness, and the name of a referring physician.

In addition, the patient is asked to provide insurance information for him- or herself and a spouse or partner. This information includes the name of the primary, secondary, and tertiary insurance carriers, name and birth date of the policyholder, the copayment, and policy and group numbers.

Coding Systems: DRG, ICD, CPT

Each of these categories of information (personal, medical, insurance) is entered into a form and becomes part of a record in a table in a database. Some of it is translated into codes before it is entered. Codes provide standardization which allows the easy sharing of information. Because codes of diagnoses and procedures are precise and universally used, one physician can recognize another's diagnoses and procedures immediately.

Standard coding systems include **DRG (diagnosis related group)**. Today, hospital reimbursement by private and government insurers is determined by diagnosis. Each patient is given a DRG classification, and a formula based on this classification determines reimbursement. If hospital care and cost exceed the prospective cost determination, the hospital absorbs the financial loss.

Services including tests, lab work, exams, and treatments are coded using **CPTs** (*Current Procedural Terminology*, 4th ed.). **ICD-9-CM** provides 3-, 4-, or 5-digit codes for more than 1,000 diseases. The ICD is the *International Classification of Diseases*, 9th ed. These coding systems make electronic claims forms easier to file because each condition or disease, each service, procedure, and diagnostic test can be identified by a widely agreed-on several-digit number. The codes are standardized, but no practice uses all of them. When a new practice is set up, only codes that relate to its specialty are entered in one of the tables of codes; these tables can always be amended. The CPT is used on the superbill or encounter form (list of diagnoses and procedures common to the practice) to identify all procedures performed by that specialty.

The Electronic Medical Record (EMR)

The information that was gathered and entered into a computer will form the patient's medical record. Slowly, the electronic medical record (EMR) is replacing the paper record. Documentation of medical conditions and treatments is going on-line.

Accounting, Using MediSoft

MediSoft is essentially an accounting program. Therefore, several definitions are required. **Charges**, **payments**, and **adjustments** are called **transactions**. A charge is simply the amount a patient is billed for the provider's service. A payment is made by a patient or an insurance carrier to the practice. An adjustment is a positive or negative change to a patient account. Transactions are organized around cases. A **case** is the condition for which the patient visits the doctor. This information is entered by the medical office staff and stored in the practice's database tables. There can be several visits associated with one case. The case can be closed when the condition is resolved. And there can be several cases (one for each diagnosis) for one patient.

Insurance

Today, many people are covered by medical insurance. Those people who are not covered either pay out-of-pocket, or seek care in the local emergency room. A **guarantor** is the person responsible for payment; it may be the patient or a third party. There are a variety of options for those with insurance. Some carriers have a **schedule of benefits**—a list of those services that the carrier will cover. This is called an **indemnity plan**. Indemnity plans are becoming less and less common, because they are **fee-for-service plans**, and therefore very expensive. The patient is never restricted to a network of providers and needs no referrals for specialists. After fulfilling a **deductible** (a certain amount the patient is required to pay each year before the insurance begins paying,) every visit to a doctor is paid for by the insurance company. The doctor, not the insurance company, determines necessary care and treatment so there is no financial reason for a health care worker to deny necessary care (Lloyd Ito, MD, http://phys-advisor.com/Insure.htm). **Managed care** (see below) also has a schedule of benefits for out-of-network providers. Managed care plans and **Preferred provider organizations (PPOs)** may require that the provider get **authorization** before a procedure is performed. This is simply permission by the insurance carrier for the provider to perform a medical procedure.

A patient with PPO insurance can seek care within an approved network of health care providers who have agreed with the insurance company to lower their charges and accept **assignment** (the amount the insurance company pays). The patient may pay a small

copayment (of five or ten dollars), the part of the charge for which the patient is responsible. The patient may choose, however, to go out-of-network and pay the provider's customary charges. The insurance company may then reimburse the patient a small amount.

There are several government insurance plans. They are administered by the federal **Health Care Financing Administration (HCFA)**, recently renamed the **Center for Medicaid and State Operations (CMS)**. Seventy-four million Americans receive their health care through government insurers—some through fee-for-service plans, some through managed care (HCFA, http://www.hcfa.gov/). According to HCFA, **Medicaid** is "jointly funded, federal-state health insurance for certain low-income and needy people. It covers approximately 36 million individuals including children, the aged, blind, and/or disabled, and people who are eligible to receive federally assisted income maintenance payments." Medicaid resembles managed care, in that the patient is restricted to a network of providers, must get a preauthorization for procedures, and needs referrals to any specialist. **Medicare** serves people age sixty-five and over and disabled people with chronic renal disorders. Medicare allows patients to choose their physicians; referrals are not needed. Some Medicare patients choose to belong to HMOs. Many people supplement Medicare with private fee-for-service plans in which they are not restricted to a network of providers and they do not need referrals to specialists. The patient is required to pay a cost-sharing amount; the provider bills the insurance for the remainder. **CHAMPVA** and **TRICARE** are federal health benefits programs that supplement medical care in the military. **Worker's Compensation** is a government program that covers job-related illness or injury.

With managed care, it is the insurance carrier that determines what treatment is necessary and pays for it. There are several forms of managed care. In managed care, patients pay a fixed yearly fee, and the insurance company pays the participating provider.

A patient who uses a health maintenance organization (HMO) pays a fixed yearly fee, and must choose among an approved network of health care providers and hospitals. The patient needs a referral from his or her primary care provider to see any specialist. If a patient goes out-of-network without the HMO's approval, the patient must pay out-of-pocket.

In a **capitated plan**, a physician is paid a fixed fee (the capitation), and the physician is paid regardless of the amount of treatment he or she provides. Some patients may seek no treatment; some may visit several times.

Claims   To receive payment for services from an uninsured patient, the practice simply bills the patient. To receive payment for services rendered to an insured patient, the practice must submit a **claim** to the insurance carrier. A claim is a request to an insurance company for payment for services. If an insurance carrier requires a treatment plan, the current version of MediSoft enables you to create one. There are many claim forms, but the most widely accepted form is the **HCFA-1500**. It is accepted by government insurers and most private plans. An **EMC (electronic media claim)** is an electronically processed and transmitted claim.

To create a claim to submit to an insurance company, the practice needs to gather certain information: the patient's condition, the physician's diagnosis, and the procedures performed in the office or hospital. The patient record can provide them with personal data, medical history, and insurance information. The provider table can supply information about the physician. Claims are submitted on paper or electronically. Practices that submit electronic claims use a **clearinghouse**—a business that collects insurance claims from providers and sends them to the correct insurance carrier. An insurance company can reject the claim, or send a check for partial or full payment. The response to a paper claim includes an **explanation of benefits (EOB)** which explains why certain services were covered and others not; an **electronic remittance advice (ERA)** accompanies the response to an EMC. The practice records the claim and applies it to the charge. It then bills the secondary insurer; the EOB from the first insurer is sent to the secondary insurer with the bill. The secondary insurer responds with a check and EOB or ERA. After the response is received from the secondary insurer, the tertiary insurance company is billed. It is only after the response is received from all of a patient's carriers that the patient is billed. This is called bucket billing or balance billing. MediSoft is structured to handle bucket billing, which is unique to the health care environment.

From the time a patient is charged for a procedure to the time when all payments have been received and credited to the patient's account, there is a sequence of accounting events that occur. **Accounts Receivable (A/R)** include any invoices or any payments from the patient or insurance carriers to the medical practice. The diagnoses and procedures relevant to a patient's visit are recorded on a **superbill** (also called an **encounter form**). A superbill is a list of diagnoses and procedures common to the practice. Superbills for each patient on a day's schedule are printed that morning or the night before. Information taken from the superbill is utilized in several MediSoft accounting reports.

Accounting Reports MediSoft provides the user with various kinds of reports that are generated on a daily, monthly, or yearly basis. Daily reports include a **patient day sheet**, a **procedure day sheet**, and a **payment day sheet**.

A patient day sheet lists the day's patients, chart numbers, and transactions. It is used for daily reconciliation. A procedure day sheet is a grouped report organized by procedure. Patients who underwent a particular procedure, such as a Blood Sugar Lab Test, are listed under that procedure. This report is used to see what procedures a health care worker is performing. It also can be used to find the most profitable procedures. A payment day sheet is a grouped report organized by providers. Each patient is listed under his or her provider. It shows the amounts received from each patient to each provider (*MediSoft Training Manual*, 6-2).

A **practice analysis report** is generated on a monthly basis, and is a summary total of all procedures, charges, and transactions (*MediSoft Training Manual*, 6-7).

A **patient aging report** is used to show a patient's outstanding payments. Current and past due balances are listed on this report based on the number of days late. For example, an account can be past due 30–60 days, 60–90 days, and over 90 (*MediSoft Training Manual*, 6-11).

The administrative and accounting tasks of a health care environment can be computerized using MediSoft. It allows the user to enter all necessary information into tables, link the information, and present it in one of the many reports it provides. Computerizing the accounting transactions allows the office to avoid being buried in paper, and keeps all accounts in an accurate, up-to-date, and well-organized structure.

Chapter Summary

- The flow of work in a medical office may start with a call from someone wanting to make an appointment. It can be recorded in MediSoft's electronic appointment book. The patient fills in a patient information form, and this information must be entered into a computer. Once the patient is seen and diagnosed, this information is also recorded electronically.
- The information collected on the patient information form includes name, address, phone, Social Security number, prior medical history, insurance information, relationship to the insured, and so on.
- Coding systems, with their affinity to both computers and the current fractured health care system, include the DRG, ICD, and CPT.
- The paper record is slowly being replaced by the electronic medical record (EMR).

- Accounting functions in a medical office include bucket (balance) billing, sending claims, recording payments and deposits. MediSoft can help streamline and structure these functions.
- There are several types of medical insurance, including Medicare, Medicaid, fee-for-service, managed care, capitated plans, health maintenance organizations, and preferred provider organizations.
- Claims are filed using a form, usually the HCFA-1500.
- MediSoft makes it easy to generate several kinds of accounting reports, such as the patient day sheet, procedure day sheet, payment day sheet, practice analysis, and patient aging reports.

Key Words

Accounts Receivable (A/R)
Adjustments
Assignment
Authorization
Balance billing
Bucket billing
Capitated plan
Case
CHAMPVA
Charges
Claim
Clearinghouse
Center for Medicaid and State Operations (CMS)
Copayment
CPT (*Current Procedural Terminology*)
Database
Database management software (DBMS)
Deductible
DRG (diagnosis related group)
Electronic medical record (EMR)
Electronic remittance advice (ERA)
EMC (electronic media claim)
Encounter form
Explanation of benefits (EOB)
Fee-for-service plans
Field

File
Guarantor
HCFA-1500
Health Care Financing Administration (HCFA)
Health maintenance organization (HMO)
Indemnity plan
ICD-9-CM (*International Classification of Diseases*)
Key field
Managed care
Medicaid
Medicare
Patient aging report
Patient day sheet
Payment day sheet
Payments
Practice analysis report
Procedure day sheet
Preferred provider organization (PPO)
Record
Relational database
Schedule of benefits
Superbill
Table
Transactions
TRICARE
Worker's Compensation

REVIEW EXERCISES

Matching Exercises

Match the term with its definition.

1. EMC (Electronic Media Claim) _____
2. Explanation of Benefits (EOB) _____
3. Health Care Financing Administration (HCFA) _____
4. Clearinghouse _____
5. Superbill _____
6. Practice analysis report _____
7. Patient aging report _____
8. Authorization _____
9. Managed care _____
10. DRG _____
11. CPT _____
12. ICD-9-CM _____
13. HCFA-1500 _____
14. Patient day sheet _____
15. Schedule of benefits _____

A. Form returned by an insurance carrier which explains why certain services were covered and others not.

B. Insurance plan in which insurance carrier determines what treatment is necessary and pays for it.

C. Formula based on this code helps determine reimbursement.

D. List of those services that the carrier will cover.

E. Codes services including tests, lab work, exams, and treatments.

F. The most widely accepted insurance form.

G. Federal agency that administers Medicaid and Medicare.

H. Report used to show a patient's outstanding payments.

I. Form on which diagnoses and procedures relevant to a patient's visit are recorded (also called an encounter form).

J. Report generated on a monthly basis; it is a summary total of all procedures, charges, and transactions.

K. Business that collects insurance claims from providers and sends them to the correct insurance carrier.

L. Electronically processed and transmitted claim.

M. 3-, 4-, or 5-digit codes for more than 1,000 diseases.

N. Permission by the insurance carrier for the provider to perform a medical procedure, that is, the insurance company deems it necessary and will cover it.

O. Report that lists the day's patients, chart numbers, and transactions.

Define the following terms:

1. Field
2. Record
3. Table
4. Database
5. Relational database

A Hands-on Introduction to MediSoft and the Appointment Book

Chapter Outline

- Learning Objectives
- The MediSoft Window
- Getting Started
  - Making An Appointment: Office Hours
  - A Note about Dates
  - The Office Hours Window
  - Making an Appointment
  - Break Entry
  - Entering Repeating Appointments
  - Finding the Next Available Time
  - Printing Appointments
  - The Patient Recall List
- Chapter Summary
- Key Words
- Review Exercises

Learning Objectives

After completing this chapter, the student will

- Be familiar with the MediSoft Window and the MediSoft toolbar
- Be familiar with the office hours window and the office hours toolbar
- Know how to change the Windows system date and the MediSoft date
- Know how to use MediSoft's office hours program

- Be able to enter appointments, breaks, and repeating appointments
- Be able to print an appointment schedule
- Be able to create a patient recall list

THE MEDISOFT WINDOW

To launch MediSoft, do the following:

- Double-click the MediSoft icon on the Windows desktop.

You will see the MediSoft window with the MediSoft title and the name of the medical practice you are working with in the title bar:

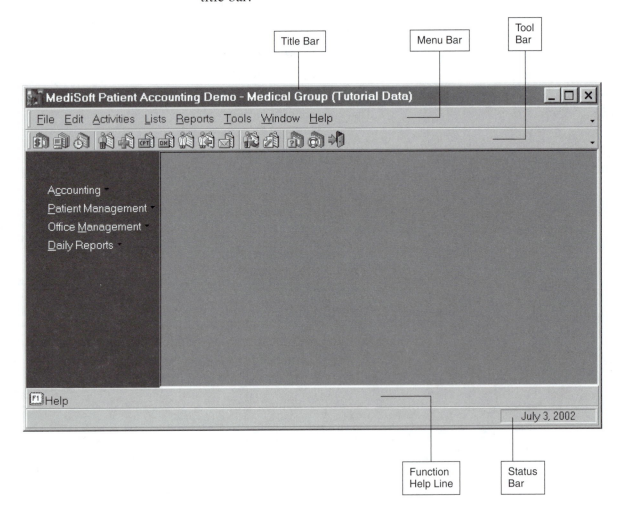

Below the title bar, the menu bar contains the names of the pull-down menus. You pull down a menu by clicking on its name.

- The **file menu** contains many options. The most commonly used options are
  - Open practice opens the database for an established practice
  - New practice sets up a new database for a new practice
  - Other options allow the user to back up and restore data, set the date, enter practice information, and perform file management tasks.

- The **edit menu** contains options to cut, copy, paste, and delete information.

- The **activities menu** contains options that allow the user to manage finances, insurance claims, and appointments, and to enter patient, diagnosis, procedure, and case information.

- The **lists menu** contains options that allow the user to enter and edit patient information, case information, procedure/payment information, adjustment codes, diagnosis, insurance and billing codes, and information on providers and referring providers.

- The **reports menu** contains a list of predefined reports, as well as custom reports and bills that the user can design. Almost all printing is done from the reports menu.

- The user can access a calculator through the **tools menu** or view the contents of a file. The tools menu also allows the user to create reports, customize menu bars, and view system information.

- The **window menu** resembles the window menu in any Windows application, allowing the user to switch between open windows (see Chapter 2).

- The user can find assistance from the MediSoft **help menu**.

Beneath the menu bar is the **MediSoft toolbar** (sometimes called the **speed bar**). The toolbar icons function in MediSoft in the same way that they function in any Windows application—they give the user fast access to common functions.

The **MediSoft sidebar** is a shortcut to accounting functions, patient and office management tasks, and daily reports.

The taskbar is at the bottom of the Windows desktop and contains the Start button, a clock, and buttons for each open application.

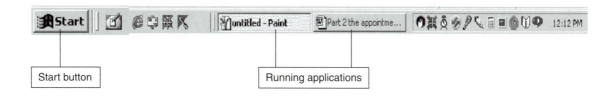

Start button   Running applications

Immediately above the taskbar is the status bar, which provides context-specific information, such as the page number and the date.

Above the status bar is the function help line (also called the shortcut bar), which contains commonly used function keys. In MediSoft, function keys work as **global commands**—commands that work from any point in the program:

- F1   Help
- F3   Save
- F4   Copy
- F6   Search
- F7   Quick Ledger
- F8   New
- F9   Edit
- F11   Quick Balance
- Shift-F3   To save a record and enter a new record.
- Other keys that function globally are the escape key to move back a screen; the tab key to move the insertion point from one field to the next; shift-tab to move the insertion point to the previous field.

The MediSoft Toolbar

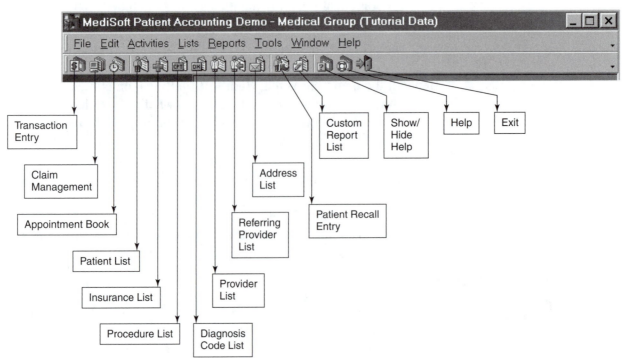

In MediSoft Advanced, there are icons for

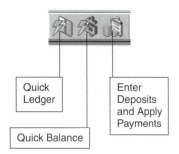

Quick Ledger

Quick Balance

Enter Deposits and Apply Payments

GETTING STARTED

Making an Appointment: Office Hours   If you (the medical office worker) are not looking at the MediSoft window, launch MediSoft by double-clicking on its icon on the desktop. The first contact between the prospective patient and a health care provider's office is the phone call to set up an appointment. The patient makes a phone call. The medical office worker who responds needs to access MediSoft's **electronic appointment book**.

Do the following:

Pull down the Activities Menu and choose appointment book or click on the appointment book icon.

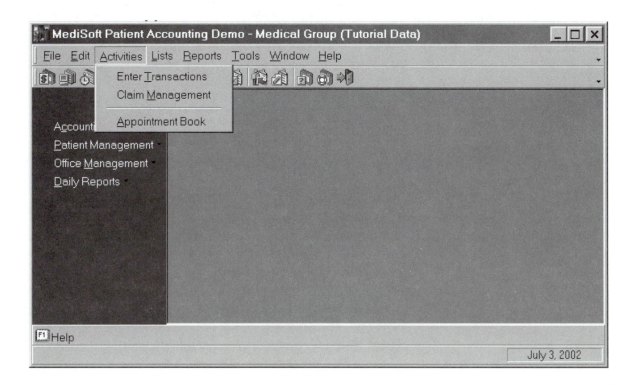

The **office hours** program and MediSoft's two-paned appointment scheduling module window will appear.

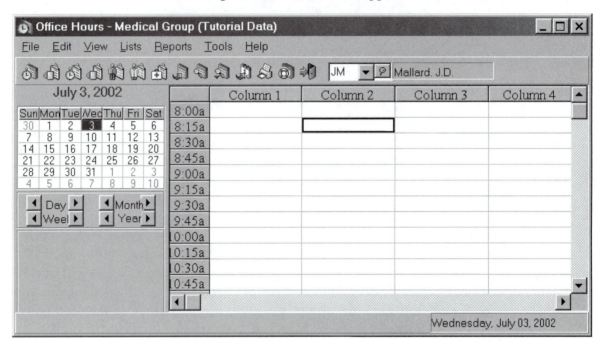

Make sure the window title says "Office Hours—Medical Group (Tutorial Data)." At the beginning we will be working with tutorial data provided by MediSoft.

Office Hours Toolbar

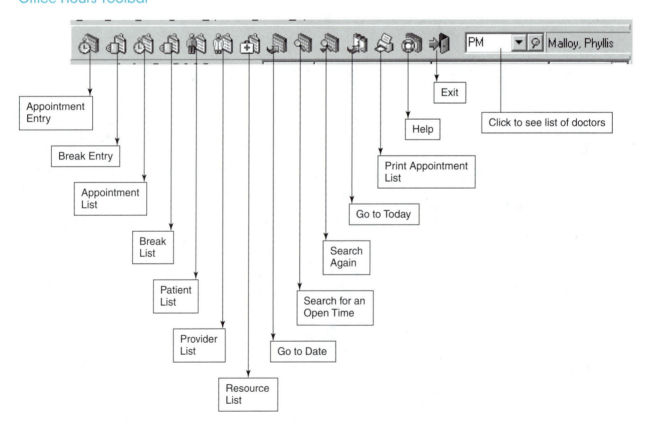

A Note about Dates MediSoft works with two dates: the **Windows system date** (today's date) on the taskbar, and the **MediSoft date** (the date the health care administrator is using) on the status bar. Because in some health care environments not all transactions are entered on the date they occurred, you need to know how to set both dates so that they are correct for the data you are entering.

To change the MediSoft date: Double-click the date on the status bar and a calendar will pop up. Change the month using the left or right arrow and change the day by clicking on the day you want. Press Enter.

To change the Windows system date: double-click the time on the taskbar and a calendar will pop up.

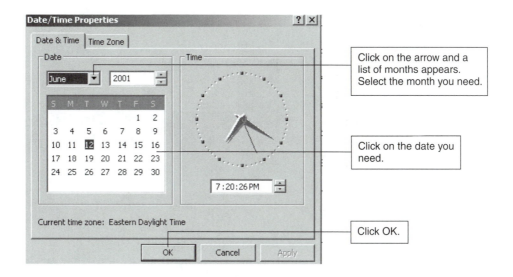

In the dialog box that opens, use the arrow in the drop-down list box to change the month and click the day you need. Click OK.

The Office Hours Window Office hours is MediSoft's scheduling software. It is sold separately from MediSoft. Office hours can be launched by double-clicking on its icon on the desktop or from within MediSoft.

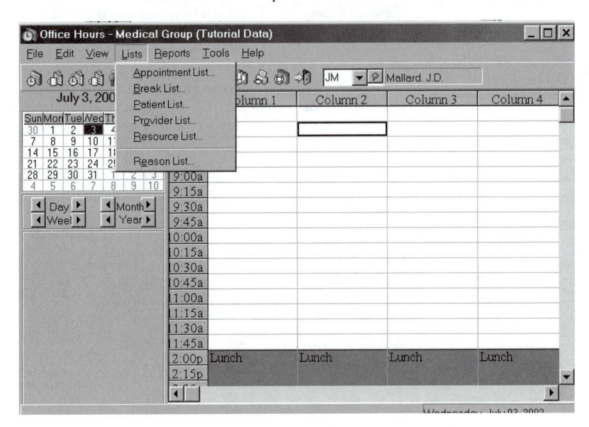

Office hours displays one month's calendar with today's date highlighted in the left pane. The right pane displays several columns for the appointments. The columns are not for multiple booking; they are meant for a health care practice with several providers. You can move the calendar backward and forward using arrow keys

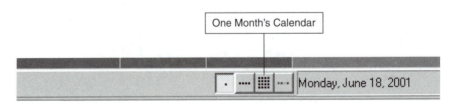. Notice that on the appointment side, blocks of time are set aside and color coded for activities that happen each day (e.g., lunch), for appointments with patients, and for other events. The appointment book toolbar contains icons that give quick access to common functions. In office hours professional icons at the bottom of the window allow the user to change the view of the calendar.

One Month's Calendar

The default choice is the current month on the left and the day's appointment calendar on the right. The next icon displays one month's calendar on the left and a week's appointment schedule with appointments and other events indicated for the provider listed on the toolbar.

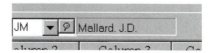

The next icon ⊞ will display the month's calendar on the left, selected; on the right every day of the month appears. On the month's calendar, you can see events indicated by color and a day with appointments surrounded by a heavy border.

Click on the ▣ icon at the bottom right of the window to return to a view of this month.

Click the down-arrow to select a provider. The following will appear:

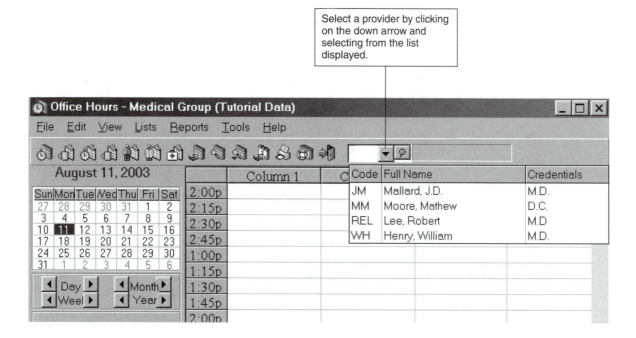

Making an Select a provider from the drop-down provider list box. Double-click
Appointment on 8:30 A.M. The following dialog box will appear.

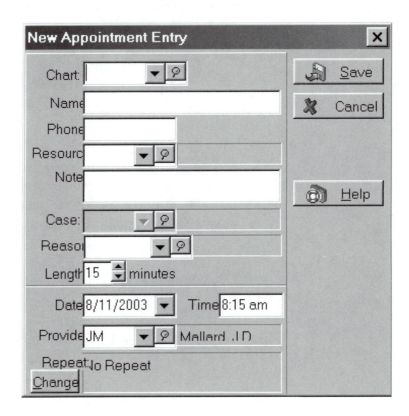

Fill in the information requested, either by using drop-down lists (for
the chart number, resource) or by entering information. MediSoft
should automatically fill in the phone number, date, time, room,
procedure code if known, and provider. Fill in the reason for the appointment by clicking on the reason drop-down list, clicking on
description, and, for this tutorial, entering backache. (Low back pain
does not appear.) Save the appointment.

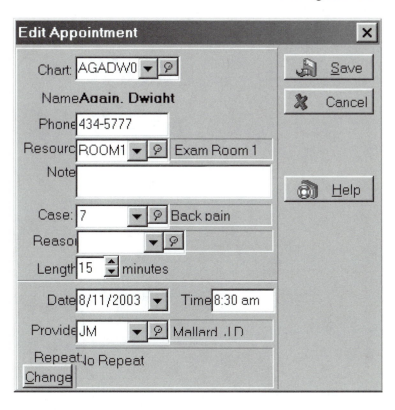

As soon as you save the appointment, it appears on the day's appointment calendar.

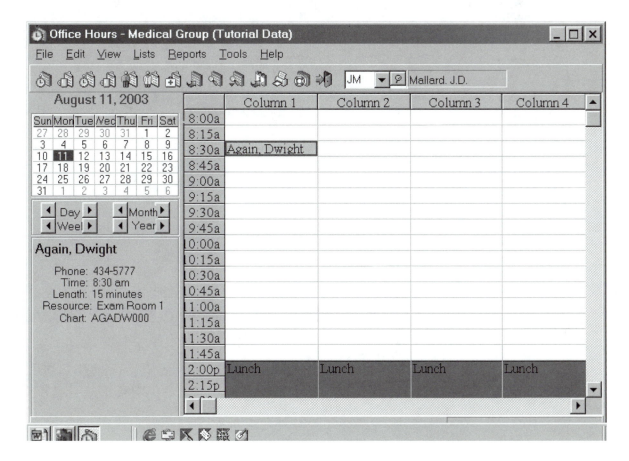

Break Entry To enter a break, for example, a coffee break that occurs every day, click on the time (4:00 P.M.) and then click on the break entry icon; the following dialog box will appear. Fill in coffee, and make sure all columns is checked:

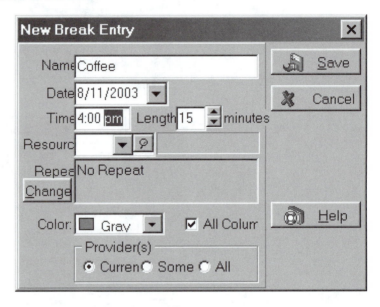

Click save and the following will appear:

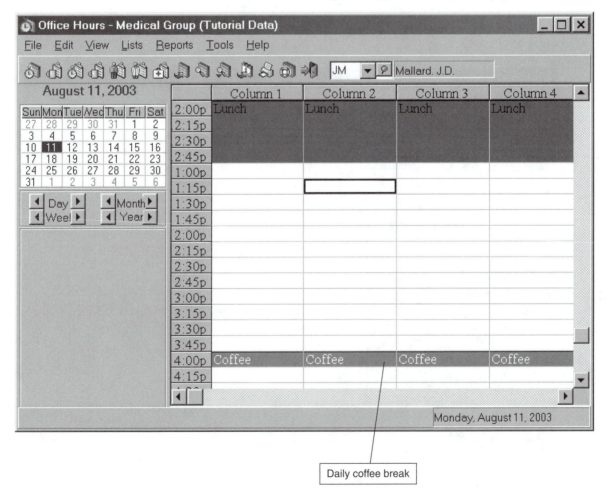

Daily coffee break

Entering Repeating Appointments

To enter **repeating appointments**, the user can click on the go to date

icon 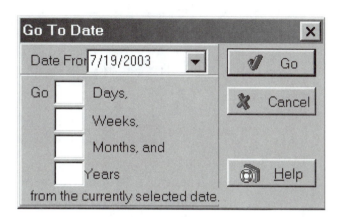 on the appointment book toolbar.

You can instruct the program to display a date that is any number of days, weeks, months, or years from today's date to make an appointment that needs to be periodically repeated. For example, if you go to a date seven days from now, that day's appointment calendar will be displayed and you can enter the appointment.

NOTE: IF A DATE NEEDS TO BE ENTERED IN THE GO TO DATE DIALOG BOX ENTER IT AS MMDDYYYY. YOU MUST USE THE FOUR DIGITS OF THE YEAR (2003, FOR EXAMPLE).

To enter a repeating appointment for Dwight Again: On July 19, as he is leaving, he might ask for an appointment in a week. Click on the go to date icon and fill in 7 in go ___ days. This will bring the calendar for July 26 onto the screen, and you can enter an appointment.

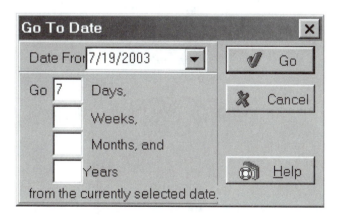

Finding the Next Available Time   If you need to find the next open appointment, you can use find open time by choosing it from the edit menu or clicking the search icon on the toolbar. Click on the search icon. A dialog box will be displayed.

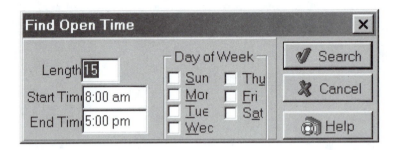

The user fills in the required information. Does this patient need an 8:00 A.M. appointment on Saturday? Click on the day (Saturday); fill in the time (8:00 A.M.); and click search. The next available open time slot on a Saturday at 8:00 A.M. will be surrounded by a heavy border. Double-click the time slot and this dialog box appears:

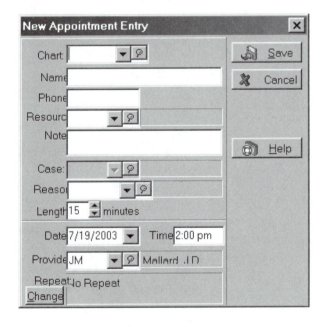

You need to fill in the chart number. If a second appointment is needed, use search again. Each time you use search again, it brings you to the next available time slot on a Saturday at 8:00 A.M.

Printing Appointments   To print the day's appointment list, click on the print icon, and then click OK.

In MediSoft Office Hours Advanced, you can easily print the **appointment grid** for the day or the week. To print the week's grid, make sure you are looking at the week's calendar. Pull down the reports menu and choose print appointment grid. The following will print:

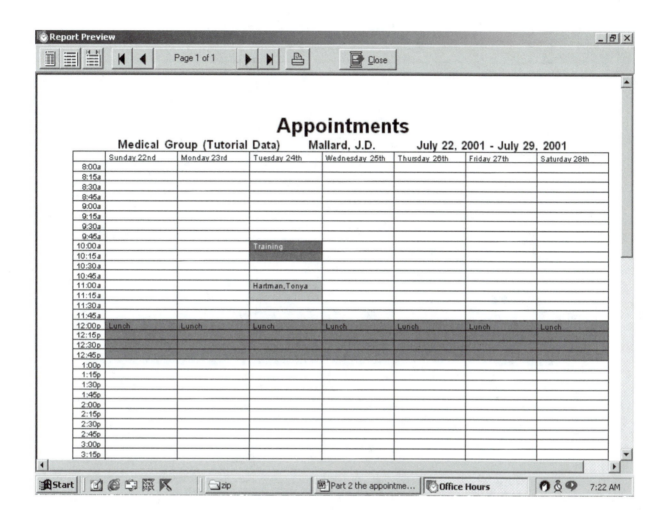

To print the day's appointment grid, make sure you are looking at the day's calendar. Pull down the reports menu and choose print appointment grid.

The following will print:

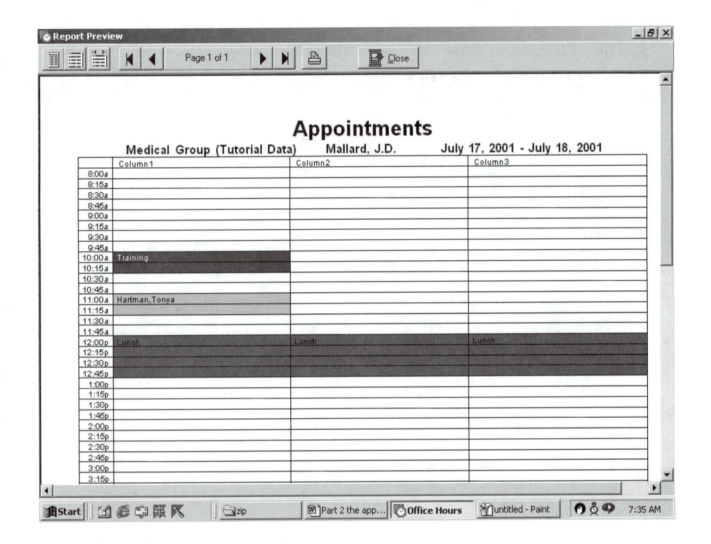

The Patient Recall List   Many patients need follow-up appointments in a week or a month or a year. MediSoft allows the user to create and edit a **patient recall list**. In the MediSoft Window (*not* the appointment book window), pull

down the lists menu and select patient recall. The following window
will appear:

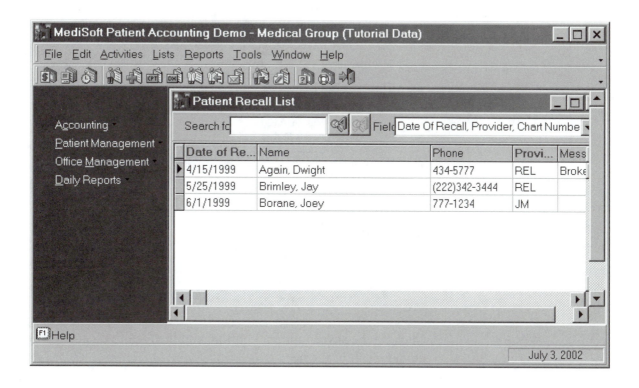

To add a patient to the recall list, click the new command button. The
following dialog box will be displayed:

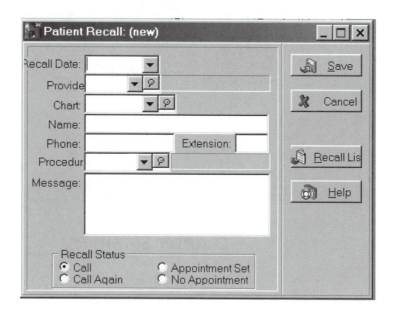

Fill in the following information by making choices from the drop-
down lists. After you select the chart number, MediSoft fills in the

patient's name and phone numbers. You need to choose the procedure and type the message. Make sure the recall status is call.

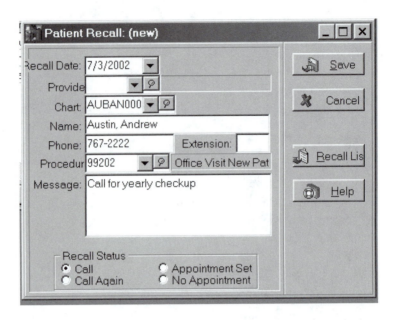

Click on the save command button, and the recall you entered appears on the recall list.

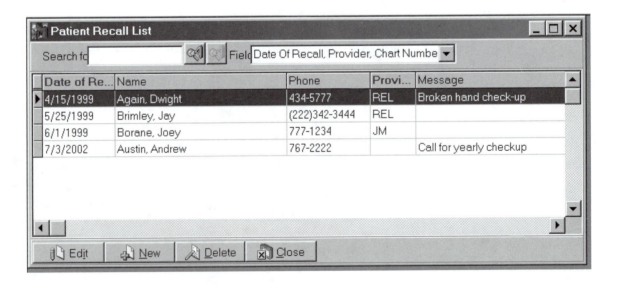

Chapter Summary

- MediSoft is launched by double-clicking on its icon on the desktop. MediSoft's window resembles any other window under Windows—with a title bar, menu bar, toolbar, and so on.
- The office hours program, which is a separate module, can be launched by double-clicking on the icon on the desktop or from within MediSoft. It is MediSoft's appointment scheduler.

- MediSoft uses two dates—the Windows system date and the MediSoft date.
- Appointments are made by choosing a provider, double-clicking the time of the appointment, and entering some information. (You may have already entered much of the information from another part of the program.)
- Breaks can be entered by clicking on the break icon and filling in the relevant information.
- Repeating appointments are made easily using search and search again.
- All appointments, breaks, and so on, are color coded on the calendar.
- MediSoft allows the user to create a patient recall list, with the dates and reasons for recall.

Key Words

Appointment grid	Office hours
Appointment list	Recall list
Electronic appointment book	Repeating appointments
Global commands	Sidebar
MediSoft date	Windows system date

REVIEW EXERCISES

Hands-on Exercises

1. Enter a coffee break every day at 10:00 A.M. Print the appointment list for today and tomorrow.

2. Enter an appointment for Dwight Again for one week from June 26, 2003 (on July 2, 2003). Print the appointment list for June 26 and July 2, 2003.

3. Choose a different provider from the provider list and make three monthly appointments (starting with today's date) for Andrew Austin. Print the appointment lists for today, one month from today, and two months from today.

4. Change the Windows system date and the MediSoft date to July 14, 2003. Make an appointment for 9:00 A.M. that day for Jay Brimley. Change the date back to today's date. Make an appointment for Jane Doe for 8:00 A.M. Print the appointment schedule for July 14, 2003, and for today.

Fill-in Questions

1. In MediSoft, _____ keys work as global commands, that is, they work from any part of the program.

2. To present information in a finished and attractive format you would first pull down the _____ menu.

Entering Patient and Case Information— A Hands-on Approach

Chapter Outline

- Learning Objectives
- Patients and Cases
- Entering and Editing Patient and Case Information
  - Jenna Green: Adding a New Patient With Medicare
  - Kathy Patel: Entering a New Uninsured Patient
  - Tonya Brown: Entering a Patient with Private Insurance
  - Jenna Green: Entering Case Information for a Patient with Medicare
  - Jenna Green: Editing Patient Information
  - Jenna Green: Adding a New Case for an Established Patient
  - Kathy Patel: Adding a Case for an Uninsured Patient
- Reports
  - Printing Patient Information
  - Printing Case Information
- A Note on Backing Up and Restoring Data
- Chapter Summary
- Key Words
- Review Exercises

Learning Objectives

Upon finishing this chapter the student will

- Understand what a case is
- Be able to enter, edit, and save patients with several types of insurance
- Be able to enter, edit, and save cases for patients
- Be able to print reports on patient information (patient face sheets and patient lists)

- Be able to print case information
- Be able to back up data on a floppy disk and restore it on another computer

PATIENTS AND CASES

Entering and Editing Patient and Case Information

When a new patient comes in for a scheduled appointment, the patient fills out forms with personal, health, insurance, and other information. The doctor enters diagnoses and procedures on the Superbill. All this information could be kept on paper. However, entering it into a computerized relational database such as MediSoft means that the information will be kept in an organized fashion and it will be easy to access. Information is entered using on-screen forms; as you save it, it becomes part of a table in a relational database. If you edit and save a record on one form, that information is changed in tables in which it appears. If information has to be entered only once, this means a great saving in time and effort. It also helps guarantee that information for a patient or case is the same everywhere it appears.

We will start by entering patient and case information. MediSoft is basically an accounting program, and although we are starting with patients and cases, some of the information we enter has a bearing on what we do later, for example, entering transactions and handling claims. An insurance carrier is the company that insures a patient. The type of insurance a patient has—Medicare or private, managed care or none—will reverberate through other functions in the program. The first patient we enter is named Jenna Green; she is over age sixty-five and therefore has federal medical insurance called Medicare. The second patient we will enter is named Kathy Patel and has just graduated from college; she is no longer under her parents' insurance policy and only has a part-time job. She cannot afford private insurance, so she has none. The last patient is Tonya Brown, whose medical insurance is one of her benefits as a full-time teacher. She has Aetna US Health Care as a **primary** and Blue Cross/Blue Shield as a **secondary insurer**. Both are preferred provider organizations (PPOs). In the exercises that follow the chapter, you will enter a record for yourself. You have managed care, that is, you belong to an HMO (health maintenance organization).

Jenna Green: Adding a New Patient with Medicare

To enter Jenna Green, launch MediSoft and pull down the lists menu and select patients/guarantors and cases.

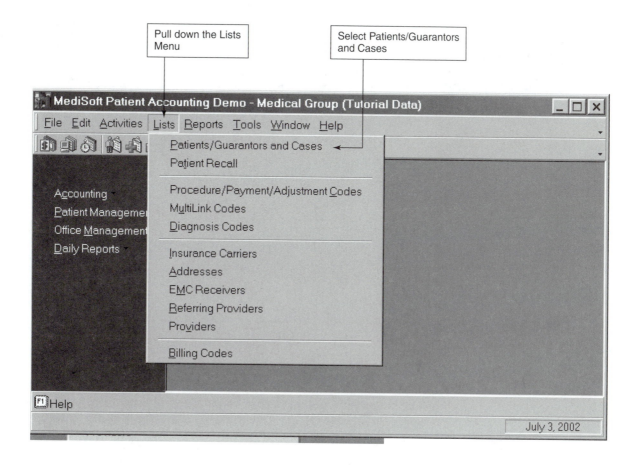

Make sure you are using the tutorial data. The following screen should appear:

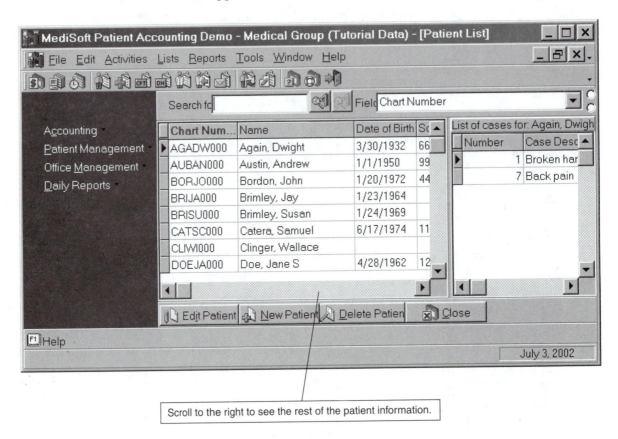

Scroll to the right to see the rest of the patient information.

The left pane contains a list of patients: chart number, name, Social Security number, date of birth, patient type, and phone number. However, to see all of this information, the user must scroll to the right. The right pane contains a list of cases for the selected patient. The selected patient is indicated by an arrowhead. **Case numbers** are assigned by MediSoft. At the top of the window are two option buttons—one for cases and one for patients. Make sure *patient* is selected. (See page 57.)

Notice that this list is sorted by **chart number**. The chart number consists of the first three letters of the patient's last name, the first two letters of the first name, and three additional digits. You can indicate which field you want to search on, although the chart number is the default. To search for a patient, enter the first three letters of the patient's last name in the Search Box, and press ENTER. Patients with chart numbers matching your search term will be displayed.

At the bottom of the window are a series of command buttons.

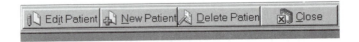

Edit patient allows you to see and change information in an existing patient's chart. New patient allows you to add a new patient. Delete patient allows you to delete a patient. If the case option button had been chosen, these command buttons would have been modified and would have allowed you to edit case, add a new case, and so on.

Do the following:

- Click on the new patient command button or press [F8]. The following dialog box appears:

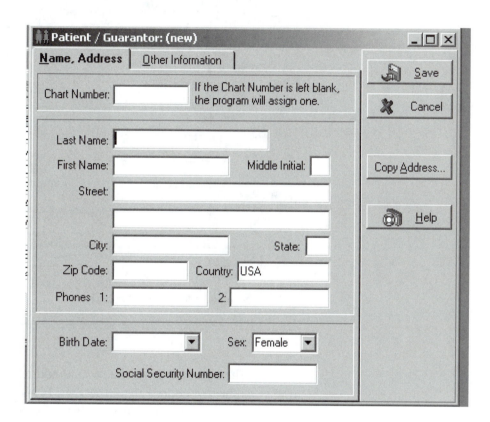

- Add the following data:
  - Tab over the chart number to the last name field.
  - With the insertion point in the last name field, type Green.
  - Tab to the first name field and type Jenna.

- Add the rest of the information (omitting chart number). *Note: Social Security numbers must be entered WITHOUT hyphens.*

In the latest version of MediSoft (v.8), the user can set the program to hyphenate social security numbers by clicking file, program options, data entry, and clicking on autoformat social security numbers.

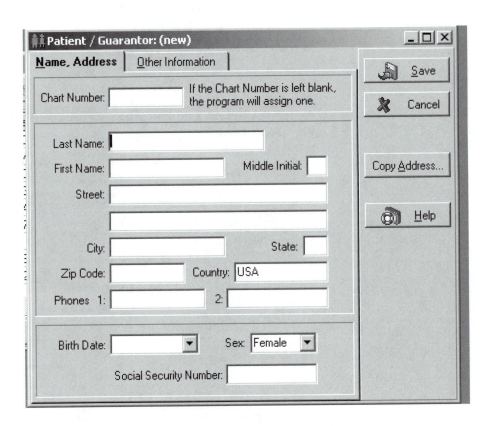

- When you tab from the second address line, MediSoft brings you to the zip code. Fill in the ZIP. If MediSoft is familiar with that ZIP (if it appears previously), MediSoft will fill in the city and state for you. Otherwise you have to fill in this information your-self. Phone numbers can be entered without parentheses and hy-phens; MediSoft automatically inserts them.

  In MediSoft Version 8, the user can enter additional information including emergency contacts and cell phone numbers.

- After completing the form, click the save command button in the upper-right corner or press [F3]. MediSoft enters a chart number for you. MediSoft also checks for duplicate Social Security numbers.

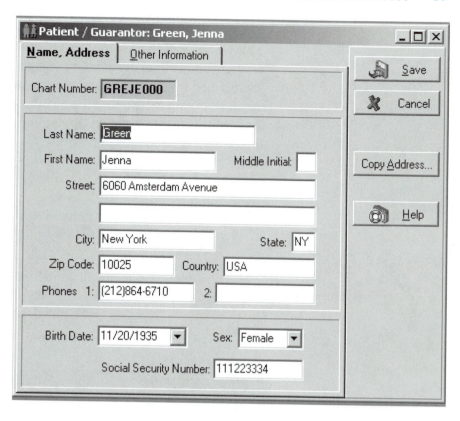

Look at the patient list. Jenna Green is correctly placed in chart number order. You could click on the other information tab and add her provider, but there are other places to add the provider. We will add it when we add her new case information.

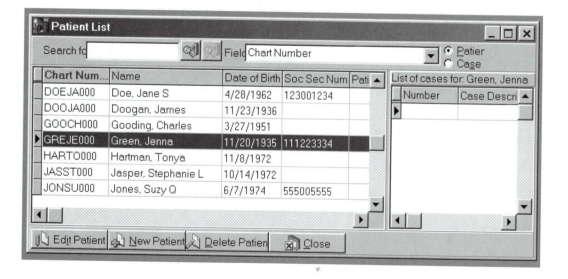

Kathy Patel: Entering a New Uninsured Patient

Kathy Patel had been using her college's health services and her parents' insurance until graduation. Because she was only able to get a job defined as part time, she has no health insurance. She calls the medical group practice to tell them she would like to become their patient, but does not make an appointment at this time. They send her the forms she needs to fill out. She returns the completed paperwork, and a medical office worker enters the information into MediSoft's patient table in the practice's database.

To enter Kathy Patel as a patient, do the following:

- Launch MediSoft.
- Pull down the lists menu and select patients/cases and guarantors.

  Press [F8] or the new patient command button.

- Fill in the following information:

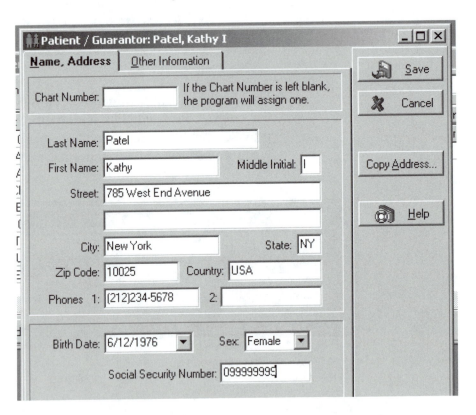

- Notice that when you enter the ZIP and press the Tab or Enter key, MediSoft fills in the city and state.
- Press the Save command button or press [F3].
- Press Enter. You will see Kathy Patel's name in the patient list.
- Open her record, and you will see the chart number MediSoft assigned.

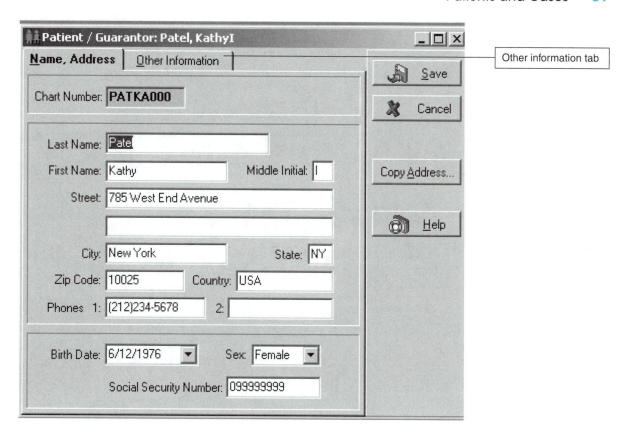

Other information tab

- Click on the other information tab and enter the information below. Make sure you enter "C" for cash. Each patient must have an assigned provider chosen from the drop-down list on the other information tab. Choose JM as the assigned provider. The signature on file check box indicates whether or not the patient's signature is on file; check it so that the patient does not have to sign each insurance form; Medicare requires this.

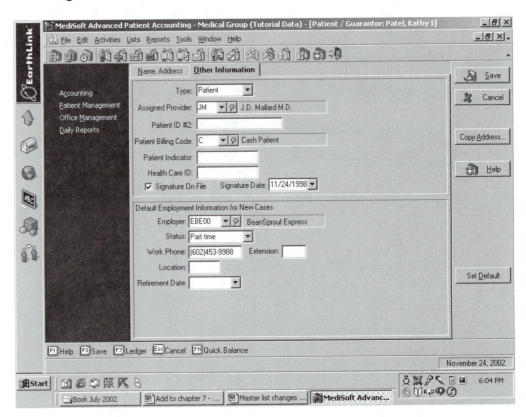

- Press the Save command button or press F3.

Tonya Brown: Entering a Patient with Private Insurance

Tonya Brown is a full-time teacher at a public school with a strong faculty union. One of the negotiated benefits is medical coverage. She had a choice of plans, and chose Aetna because all the health care providers she used were in the Aetna network of providers, as was the better hospital in her neighborhood. As a secondary insurer, she selected Blue Cross/Blue Shield.

Enter Ms. Brown in the patient table by doing the following:

- Launch MediSoft and pull down the lists menu.
- Choose patients/cases and guarantors.
- Press the new patient command button or press F8 and fill in the following information. When you click on save or press

  F3, MediSoft will assign a chart number (BROTA000).

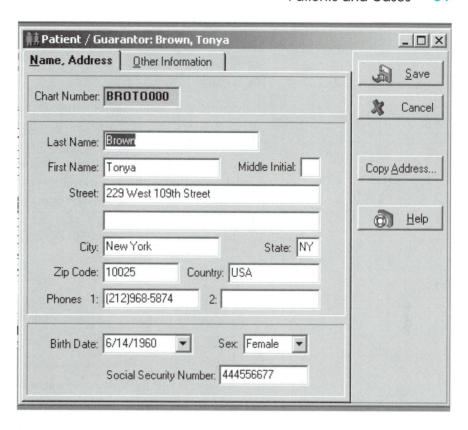

• Click the other information tab and fill in the following:

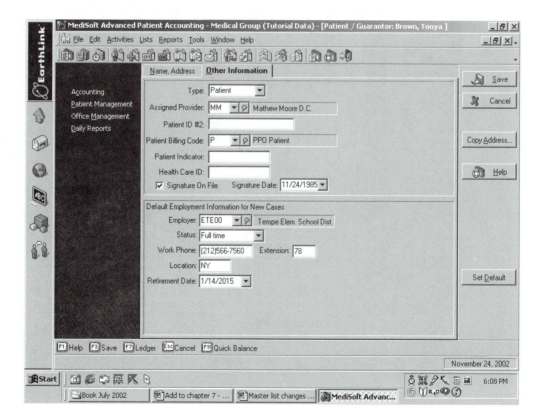

- Press the save command button or press the F3 function key.

Jenna Green: Entering Case Information for a Patient with Medicare

Remember that Jenna called to make an appointment. Her reason for seeing the health care provider is called a case. There can be more than one visit associated with one case. For example, a child with an ear infection needs to make two visits. As long as the underlying **condition** remains the same, many visits constitute one case. And of course there can be many different cases associated with one patient.

To add a new case for Jenna, do the following:

- Click on Jenna's record in the patient list.
- Make sure the case option button is chosen. Jenna's record will no longer look selected, but there will be an arrowhead next to it.
- Click the new case command button or press the F8 function key.

  You will see the following tabbed dialog box with the personal tab chosen and the name and guarantor filled in.

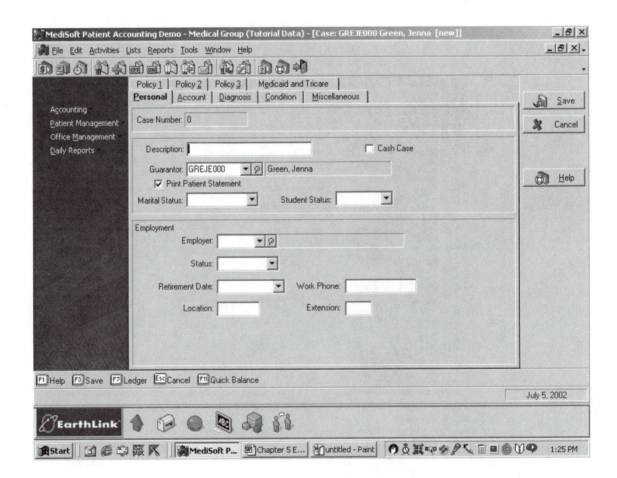

• Fill in the rest of the information.

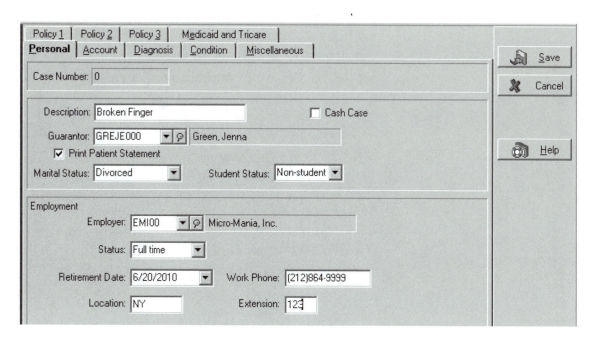

• Click on save or press the F3 Function key; you will be told that there is no **assigned provider**.
• Click on the account tab.

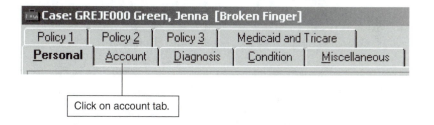

• Click on account tab.

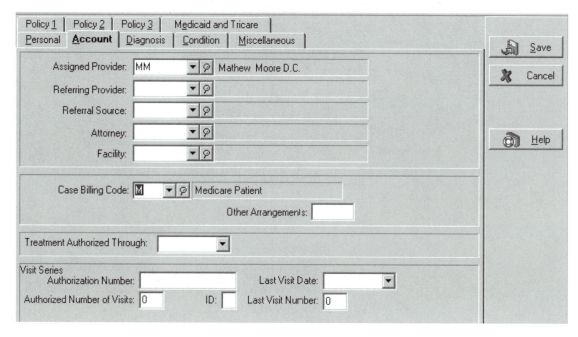

- Click the down arrow in the assigned provider drop-down list box and select Jim Mallard.
- Click the down-arrow in the **case billing code** drop-down list box and choose "M" for Medicare.
- Click on the save command button or press the F3 function key.

> NOTE: BE SURE TO SAVE EACH PAGE OF A TABBED DIALOG BOX IMMEDIATELY AFTER YOU FILL IN THE INFORMATION. IF YOU ARE BROUGHT BACK TO THE LIST OF PATIENTS/CASES AND GUARANTORS, CLICK ON THE PATIENT YOU ARE ENTERING AND CLICK THE EDIT PATIENT COMMAND BUTTON. IF YOU ARE ENTERING A CASE, CLICK ON THE PATIENT, CLICK ON THE CASE OPTION BUTTON, AND CLICK ON THE EDIT CASE COMMAND BUTTON.

- Click on the condition tab and the following dialog box appears:

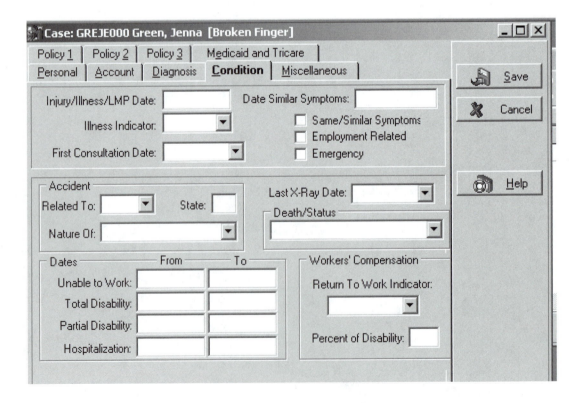

- Fill in the information by typing in the date, and making choices from drop-down lists for the other fields. Do not fill in anything in fields that are blank.

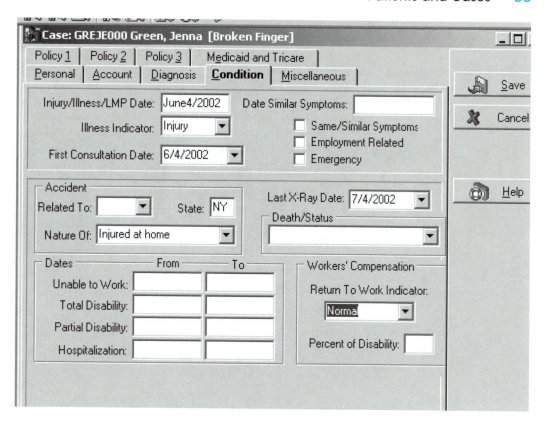

- Press the save command button or press the F3 function key.
- Click on the diagnosis tab and fill in the diagnosis by clicking on the down-arrow in the default diagnosis 1 drop-down list box. You will have to scroll through the choices until you see "broken finger." Click on broken finger. MediSoft fills in the code.
- Under Allergies and Notes, type "Allergic to aspirin."
- Click the save command button or press the F3 function key.

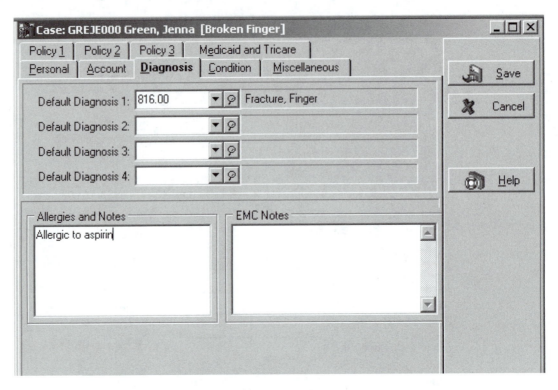

Jenna Green: Editing Patient Information

Once a patient is entered in the system, it is possible to change patient information. If Jenna calls to say she has moved to a new address, do the following:

- Pull down the lists menu.
- Choose patients/guarantors and cases.
- In the dialog box that opens, choose the patient option button.

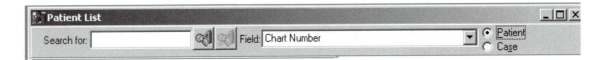

- Click on Jenna's record.

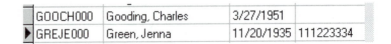

- Click on the edit patient command button.

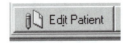

- Enter the new address: 123 Broadway.

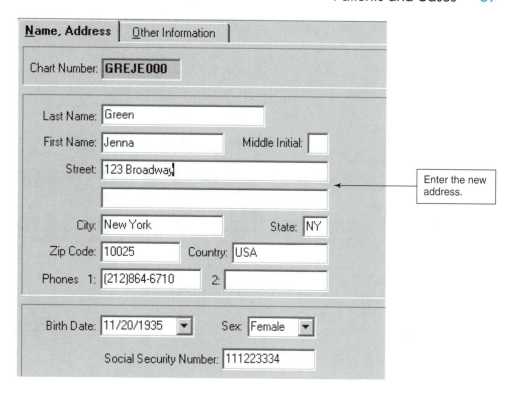

Enter the new address.

- Click the save command button or press the F3 function key.

Jenna has one follow-up appointment for her broken finger (two appointments for one case).

Jenna Green: Adding a New Case for an Established Patient

Several weeks later Jenna woke up with a sore throat and called the health care provider. She made an appointment. Pull down the patient list, and make sure it is sorted by chart number. On the patient list, it is easy to find a patient by typing in the first three letters of the patient's last name. Enter GRE as a search term.

Enter GRE

The patient list is sorted by chart number, so that you can search for a chart number.

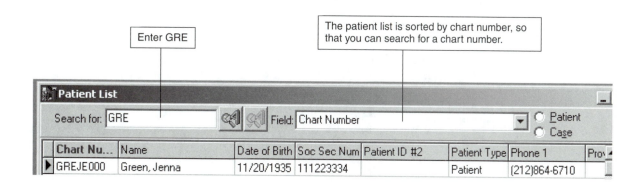

Once you have found the patient, do the following:

- Choose the case option button. You could click on new case. However, if you did that you would have to reenter much information that remains the same.
- Click on copy case.
- Change the information that needs to be changed.

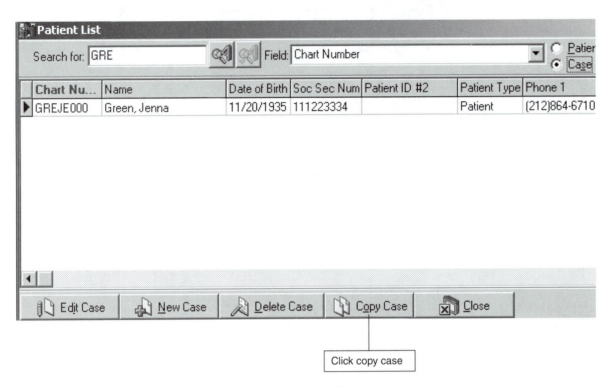

Click copy case

The following dialog box will appear:

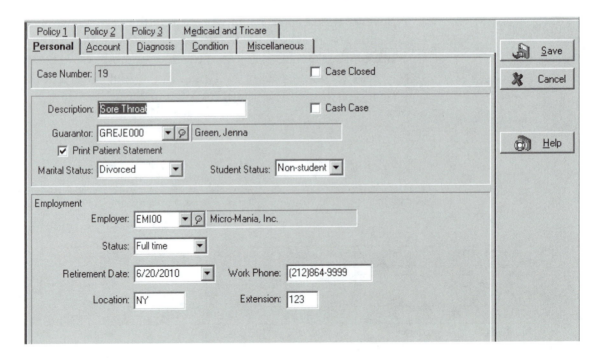

Do the following:

- Change the description to sore throat by dragging the mouse over broken finger to select the text and entering the new information: sore throat.

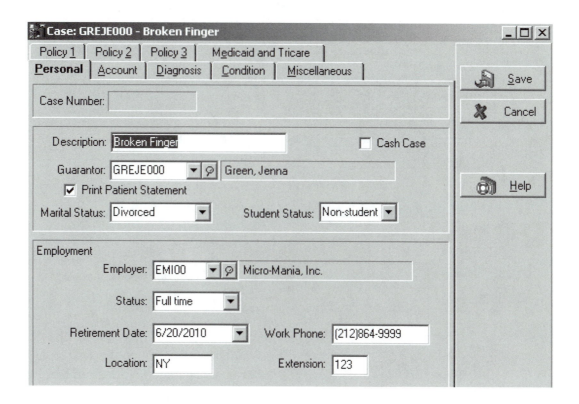

The case number is entered by MediSoft. All other information on this screen remains the same.

- Click on the diagnosis tab. The following screen appears:

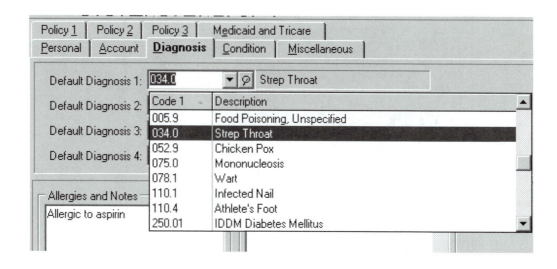

- Click the down-arrow in the default diagnosis 1 drop-down list box and select strep throat.
- Click the condition tab and the following page of the dialog box is displayed:

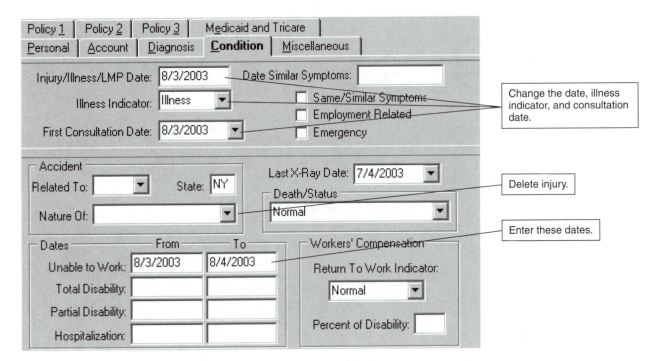

- Change the date to 8/3/2003 and choose illness from the drop-down illness indicator list. Enter the first consultation date as 8/3/2003. Enter dates unable to work from 8/3/2003 to 8/4/2003.
- Click the save button or press the F3 function key.

Look at the patient list. Click on Jenna Green. Click on patient. You will see two cases associated with Jenna Green's name.

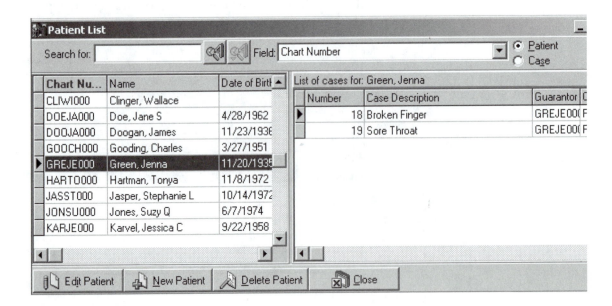

Kathy Patel: Adding a Case for an Uninsured Patient

Kathy Patel was jogging when she tripped and sprained her ankle. She called the practice to make an appointment. Remember that she had already filled out the patient information form and that that data had been entered. To add the case information, do the following:

- Pull down the lists menu and choose patients/cases and guarantors.
- Select Kathy's record.
- Click on the case option button.
- Click on the New Case Command 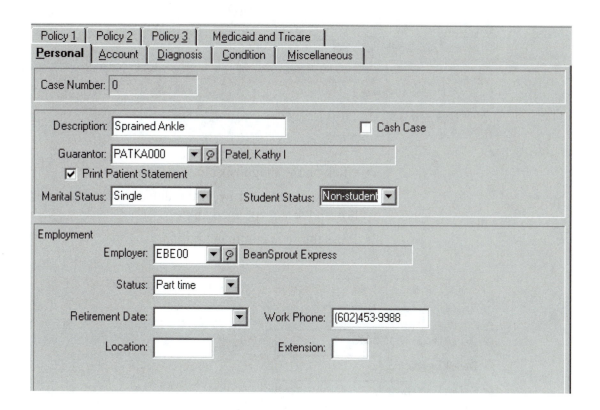 button and fill in the following information on the personal page of the dialog box:

- Press the save command button.

- Click on the account tab and make sure the following information is entered:

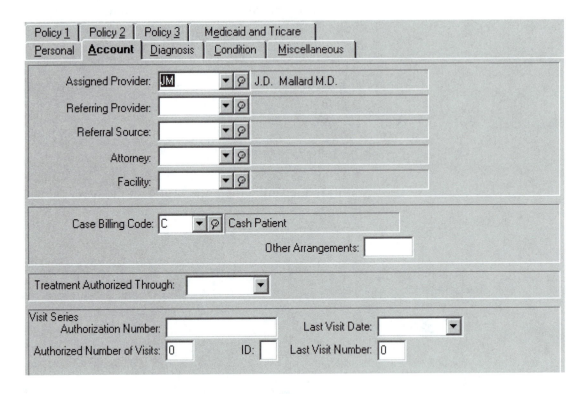

- Click on the diagnosis tab.
- Click the down-arrow in the default diagnosis 1 drop-down list box and select sprained ankle.
- Press the save command button.

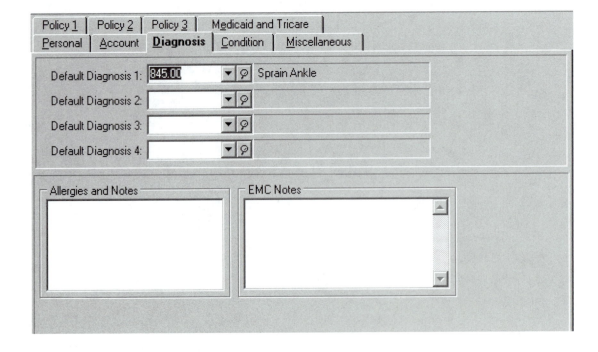

- Click on the condition tab and fill in the following information:

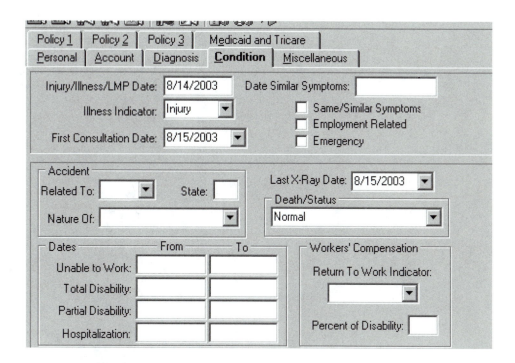

- Press the save command button.

Because she has no insurance, that is all the information you need to fill in.

In the version of MediSoft currently in use, you are able to enter treatment plans. Pull down the lists menu and select patient treatment plans, select the patient's chart number from the drop-down list, and a list of his or her plans will be displayed. Click the new plan command button, and in the dialog box that opens, fill in the description, for example, chest pains, and click OK. Click on procedure, click the new procedure command button, and select electrocardiogram-interp from the drop-down list box; enter the description (electrocardiogram-interp) and enter the amount as $45.00. Click OK. Your plan will be displayed on the treatment plans list.

REPORTS

Printing Patient Information   In MediSoft (Version 7), most printing is done from the reports menu. In MediSoft Advanced (Version 8), you can also print from almost any window. To print a list of patients:

• Pull down the Reports menu and select **custom report** list.

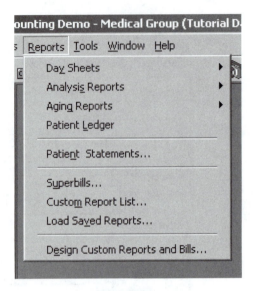

The following list will be displayed:

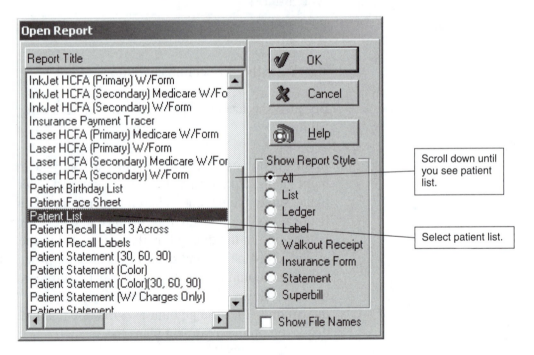

Scroll down until you see patient list.

Select patient list.

• Scroll down until you see patient list.
• Select patient list.
• Click OK.

- In the print report where? dialog box, make sure preview the report on the screen is selected and click start.

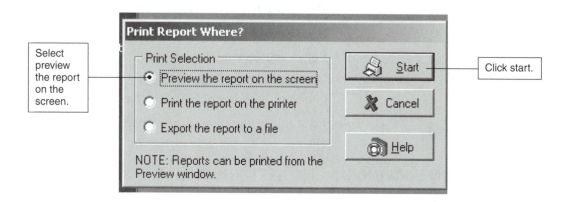

The next screen asks for the range of chart numbers you want to print.

- Leave the range blank to print all records.

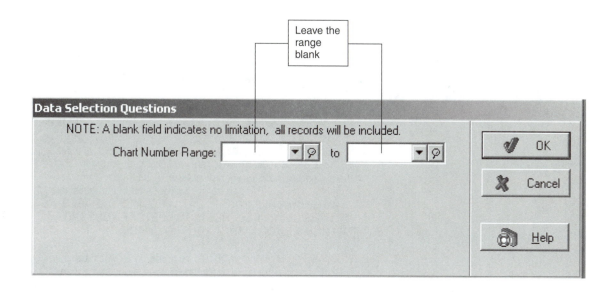

- Click OK. A **patient list** will appear on the screen. Do not print it at this time. Print it only after completing all the Hands-on Exercises at the end of the chapter. To print, you will click on the print icon.

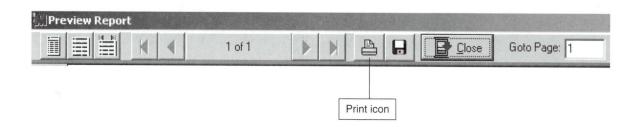

Printing Case   The steps to print case information are very similar to the steps for
Information   printing patient information.

- Pull down the reports menu and select custom report.
- Select patient face sheet.
- Select preview the report on the screen.
- In the data range dialog box, enter the chart number for Jenna Green in both boxes. Preview the report.
- Print the report only after completing the Hands-On Exercises.

A NOTE ON BACKING UP AND RESTORING DATA

If you need to carry your MediSoft database from one computer to another, you can **back up** your files on a floppy disk and **restore** them on another computer. You can back up your data by pulling down the file menu, and selecting backup data, or by waiting until you exit MediSoft, so that you are sure you back up the latest version of your files.

When you exit Medisoft (file, exit, or click on the close button in the top right of the window), the following dialog box is displayed:

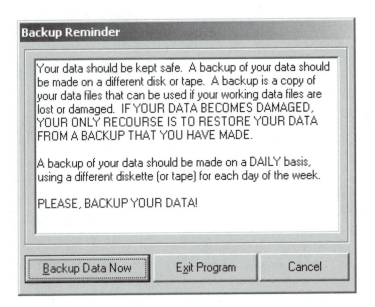

You may just exit the program. However, you may choose to back up your data. (See Chapter 11, on backing up data.)

To make a backup copy of your data, click on the backup data now command button. The following dialog box appears. Enter a:\ as the destination file path.

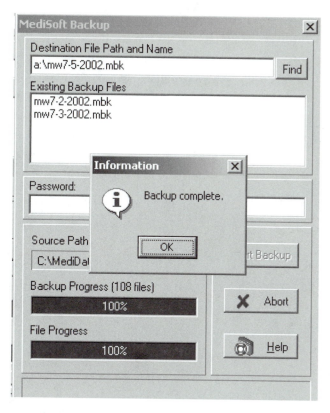

Make sure you have a disk in the A: drive and click the A: option button. Click start backup. When MediSoft has finished backing up your data, the following window is displayed:

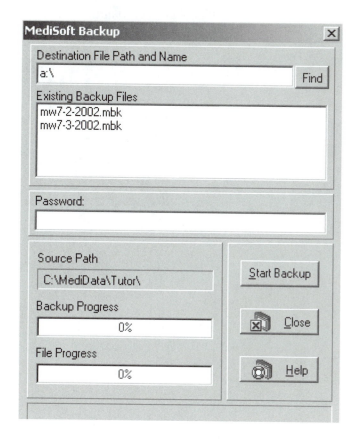

Click OK.

To access the data on the disk, for example, to work on it on another computer, you cannot simply open My Computer, and click on the A: drive. It will not open the backup file. Instead, pull down the file menu and select restore data.

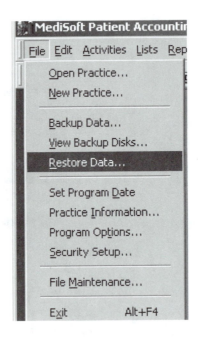

The following warning will appear:

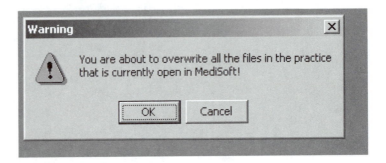

If you click OK, the following dialog box is displayed:

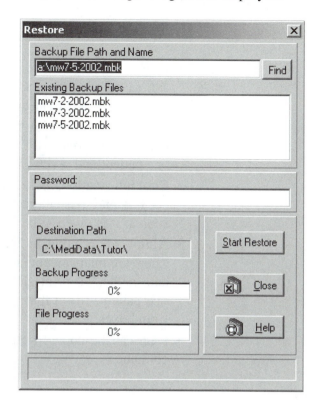

Make sure A: is chosen as the source disk and click the start restore command button. When prompted that MediSoft is about to restore the file, click OK.

When the restore is finished, the following message is displayed on the screen.

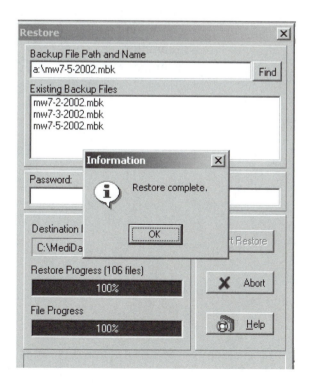

Chapter Summary

- Patients with different types of insurance can be entered, edited, and saved on a patient form. As the records are saved, they become part of a patient list.
- A case is the condition for which a patient seeks treatment from a health care provider. There can be several cases associated with one patient and several visits associated with one case.
- Case information, including condition, diagnoses, insurance carriers 1, 2, and 3, is entered in a many paged (tabbed) dialog box. As soon as it is saved, it becomes part of a case record for a patient.
- Almost all printing in MediSoft is done from the reports menu. There are many custom reports. You choose a report and fill in the data range. To print all patients leave the range blank. To print one patient, fill in that patient's chart number in both the to and from boxes.
- Data can be copied onto a floppy disk and restored on another computer.

Key Words

Assigned provider
Back up
Case numbers
Chart number
Custom reports
Condition
Guarantor
Insurance carrier

Patient billing code
Patient face sheet
Patient list
Primary insurer
Restore
Secondary insurer
Tertiary insurer
Visit

REVIEW QUESTIONS

1. MediSoft creates chart numbers using the first three letters of the patient's last name followed by the first two letters of the patient's first name, followed by three digits (000 if the patient is the only one with that name).

   What chart numbers would MediSoft create for the following patients?

   Loretta Washington _____

   Jennifer Ramirez _____

   David Cohen _____

   Edith Shah _____

   Debby Chin _____

2. Define the following terms.

   Case _____

   Carrier _____

   Medicare _____

   Guarantor _____

REVIEW EXERCISES

BE SURE TO SAVE EACH PAGE OF A TABBED DIALOG BOX BY PRESSING [F3] OR CLICKING ON THE SAVE COMMAND BUTTON IMMEDIATELY AFTER YOU FILL IN THE INFORMATION. YOU WILL BE BROUGHT BACK TO THE LIST OF PATIENTS/CASES AND GUARANTORS. CLICK ON THE PATIENT YOU ARE ENTERING AND CLICK EDIT PATIENT. IF YOU ARE ENTERING A CASE, CLICK ON THE PATIENT, CLICK ON THE CASE OPTION BUTTON, AND CLICK ON EDIT CASE.

1. Enter a new patient with your own first and last names by doing the following:
   a. Launch MediSoft by double-clicking on its icon.
   b. Pull down the lists menu.
   c. Select patients/guarantors and cases.
   d. Make sure the patient option button is selected.
   e. Click on the new patient command button or press [F8].
   f. In the dialog box that opens, fill in your own information: your last and first names, address, date of birth, and so on.
   g. Click on the other information tab. Enter JM as your provider.
   h. Save the record. Look at the patient list. Your name should be correctly placed in chart number order.

2. Add a case for yourself; you belong to a CIGNA HMO. Do the following:
   a. Pull down the lists menu and select patients/guarantors and cases.
   b. Select yourself as the patient by clicking on your record.
   c. Click on the case option button. Notice that your record is no longer selected, but there is a pointer next to it.
   d. Click on the new case command button or press ⬚. Note that MediSoft enters a case number.

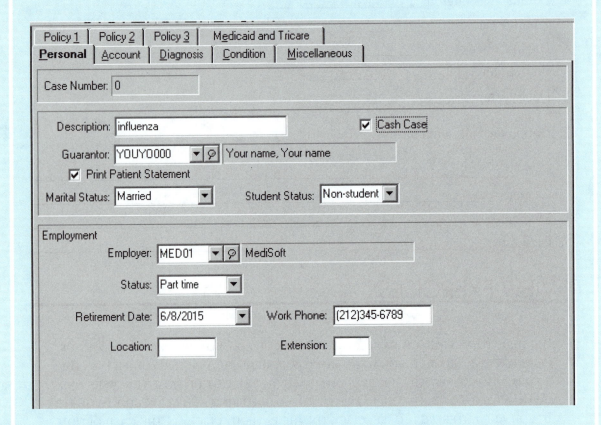

Of course your chart number will be made up of the letters of your last and first names.

e. Make sure you click on the insurance tab and fill in the following. Your insurance is CIGNA—an HMO.

Personal	Account	Diagnosis	Condition	Miscellaneous

Policy 1 | Policy 2 | Policy 3 | Medicaid and Tricare

Insurance 1: `CIG00` ▼ 🔎 Cigna

Policy Holder 1: `YOUYO000` ▼ 🔎 Your name, Your name

Relationship to Insured: `Self` ▼

Policy Number: `232455`

Group Number: `54`

Policy Dates
Start: `6/1/2000` ▼
End: ▼

☐ Assignment of Benefits/Accept Assignment

☐ Capitated Plan

Annual Deductible: `0`

Copayment Amount: `0.00`

Insurance Coverage Percents by Service Classification   A: `80`

f. Click on the save command button.

g. Click on the accounts tab. Make sure the billing code is "H" for HMO and save the record.

h. Click on the diagnosis tab.

i. Click on the down arrow in the default diagnosis 1 drop-down list box. Scroll down until you see influenza. Click on it. And save the record.

j. Click on the condition tab.

k. Fill in the illness/injury and first consultation dates as today's date.

l. Click on the down-arrow in the illness indicator drop-down list box and select illness.

m. Click on the down-arrow in the death/status drop-down list box and select normal.

n. In unable to work, fill in today's date in the from date, and tomorrow's date as the to date.

o. Save the record. Look at the patient list. Your name has a case associated with it.

3. Enter a New Case for Tonya Brown.

   a. Her personal information in the case dialog box is as follows:
- The guarantor and case number are filled in by MediSoft. You may have to fill in employer and employment information.
- Description: Bronchitis
- Marital Status: Single

- Student Status: Nonstudent
- Save the record.

b. On the account page, fill in her case billing code as "H" for HMO patient and treatment authorized through as 8/1/2003. Save the record.

c. On the diagnosis page, select bronchitis as the default diagnosis 1. Save the record.

d. On the condition page, fill in 6/12/2003 as the illness date, the illness indicator as illness, and the first consultation date as 6/14/2003. Tonya will be unable to work from 6/12/2003 to 6/21/2003. Save the record.

e. On the policy 1 page, choose Aetna from the insurance 1 drop-down list displayed when you click on the drop-down arrow in the insurance 1 list box and 9/1/1982 as the start date of the policy. Save the record.

f. On the policy 2 page, choose Blue Cross/Blue Shield as the secondary insurer. Enter the policy number, group number, and policy date information below.

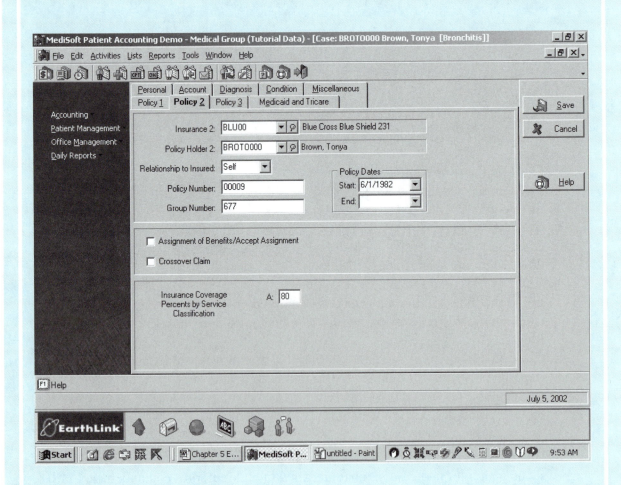

4. Print the patient list and the patient face sheets for yourself, Jenna Green, Kathy Patel, and Tonya Brown. See pages 72–75, for printing instructions. Remember, when you print the patient face sheets, each patient has to be printed as a separate report. Enter the chart number of the patient you want to print in the from and to drop-down list boxes.

Patient List

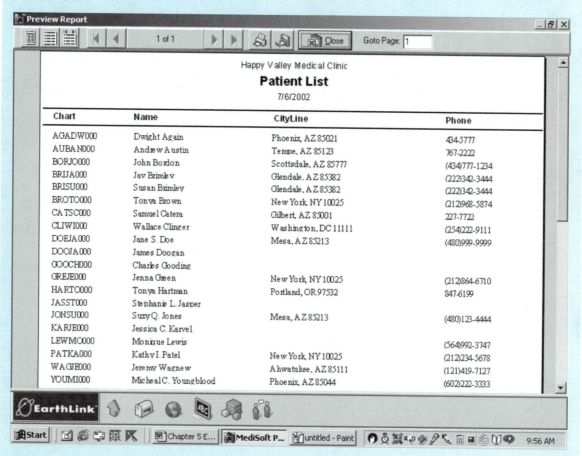

Patient Face Sheet Jenna Green

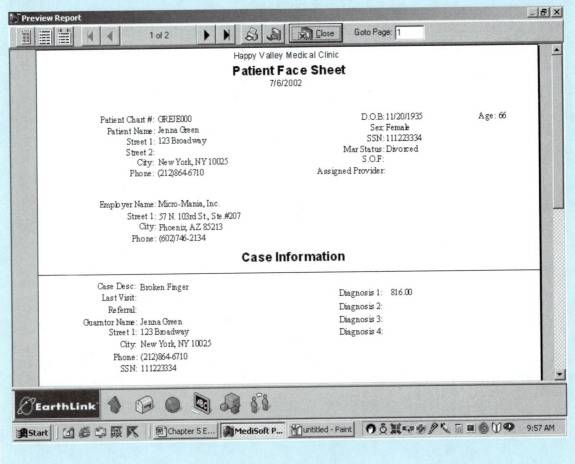

Kathy Patel's Patient Face Sheet

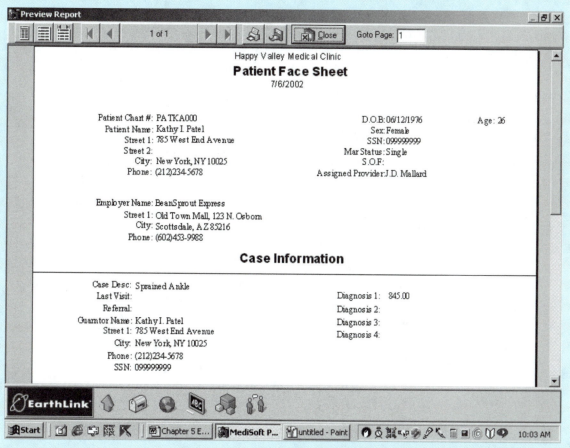

Your Patient Face Sheet

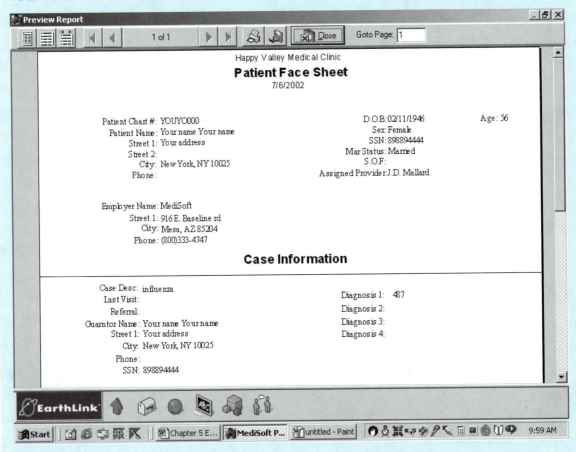

Happy Valley Medical Clinic
Patient Face Sheet
7/6/2002

Patient Chart #: YOUYO000
Patient Name: Your name Your name
Street 1: Your address
Street 2:
City: New York, NY 10025
Phone:

D.O.B: 02/11/1946   Age: 56
Sex: Female
SSN: 898894444
Mar Status: Married
S.O.F:
Assigned Provider: J.D. Mallard

Employer Name: MediSoft
Street 1: 916 E. Baseline rd
City: Mesa, AZ 85204
Phone: (800)333-4747

Case Information

Case Desc: influenza
Last Visit:
Referral:
Guarntor Name: Your name Your name
Street 1: Your address
City: New York, NY 10025
Phone:
SSN: 898894444

Diagnosis 1:   487
Diagnosis 2:
Diagnosis 3:
Diagnosis 4:

6

An Introduction to Transaction Entry and Claim Management

Chapter Outline

- Transaction Entry
  - Entering Transactions: Charges, Payments, and Adjustments (Old Style)
- Claim Management
  - Printing a Primary Claim Summary
- Entering Deposits
- Quick Ledger and Quick Balance
- New Style Transaction Entry
- Chapter Summary
- Key Words
- Review Exercises

Learning Objectives

Upon completion of this chapter, the student will

- Be able to define transaction
- Understand transaction entry (old and new style)
- Be able to enter, edit, and apply payments and charges and save this information
- Understand claim management
- Know how to create and print claims
- Check the status of claims
- Understand how to apply payments to charges
- Be able to print a deposit list report
- Know how to check on a patient's billing status using quick ledger and quick balance
- Understand new style transaction entry

TRANSACTION ENTRY

Once a patient is established and has at least one case associated with her/him, transactions must be entered and claims sent to the insurance carrier (or bills to the patient).

A transaction can be a charge to a patient's account, a payment made by insurance or the patient, or an adjustment to the patient's account (adjustments are discussed in the next section).

Entering Transactions: Charges, Payments, and Adjustments (Old Style)

In MediSoft Version 7, to enter a transaction old style (that is, in the same way as in Version 6), pull down the file menu and choose program options, click on the data entry tab and click on use old style transaction entry.

In MediSoft Version 7 (old style transaction entry), charges are entered in one window and payments entered in another window. In Version 7 (new style transaction entry), charges and payments are entered in one two-paned window. In Version 8, charges and payments must be entered in one two-paned window.

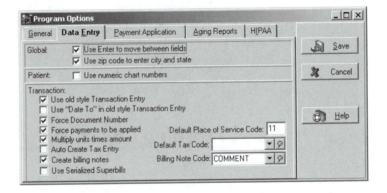

Then, do the following:

- Pull down the activities menu and choose enter transactions. The following dialog box appears:

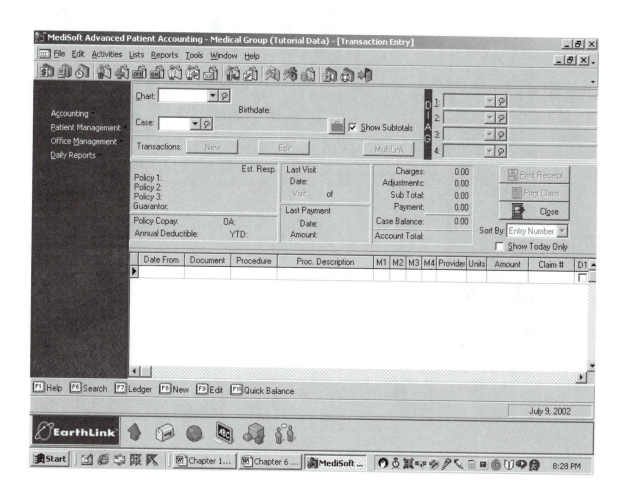

- Pull down the chart drop-down list box and select Jenna Green's chart number, and pull down the case number drop-down list box and select strep throat as the case. Your dialog box should appear similar to the following:

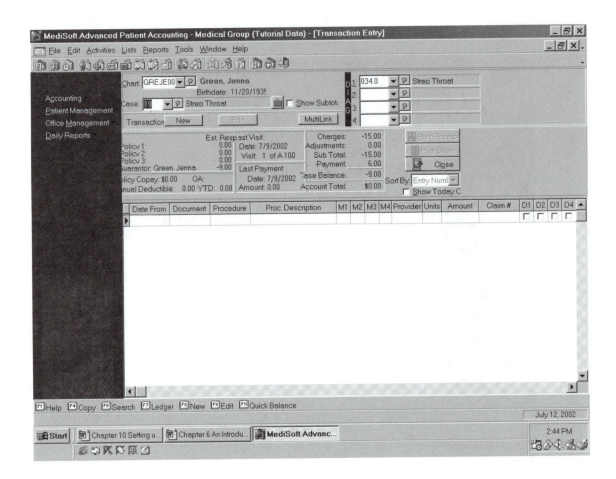

- Notice that you filled in only the chart number, which links with patient information, and the case number, which links with case, procedure, and charge information. MediSoft fills in much of the rest of the information for you, taking it from other tables in the database.

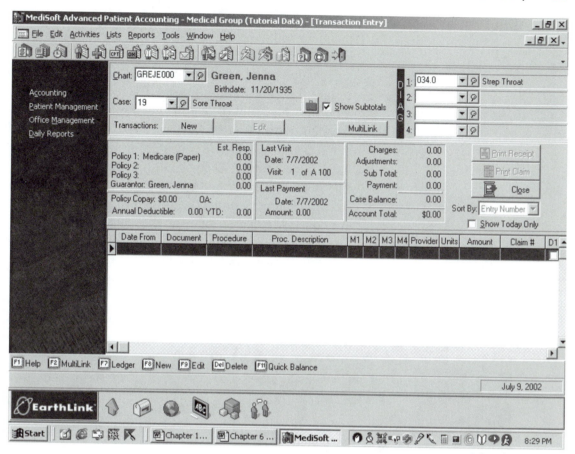

- Click new (you are entering a new transaction) and a tabbed dia-log box will appear.

- Click the charge tab and fill in the **procedure**, and the kind of payment (e.g., check, cash). Make sure the date is correct; it should be the date the procedure was performed. MediSoft assigns a document number based on this date. You fill in the procedure. Each procedure has a CPT code. Some codes also have modifiers made up of one or two digits. Modifiers allow a more detailed description of the procedure. Note the multilink command button. Multilink codes are groups of CPT codes that relate to one activity. Using multilink codes saves time. MediSoft fills in the price charged by the practice, and the amount allowed by the insurance company for the procedure (called the Allowed Amount). Medicare, for example, allows $9.00 for a strep culture for which the practice charges $15.00. The $6.00 is an adjustment to the patient's account.

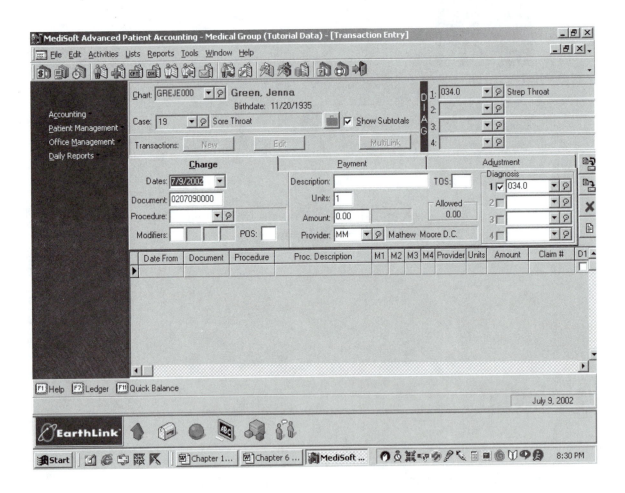

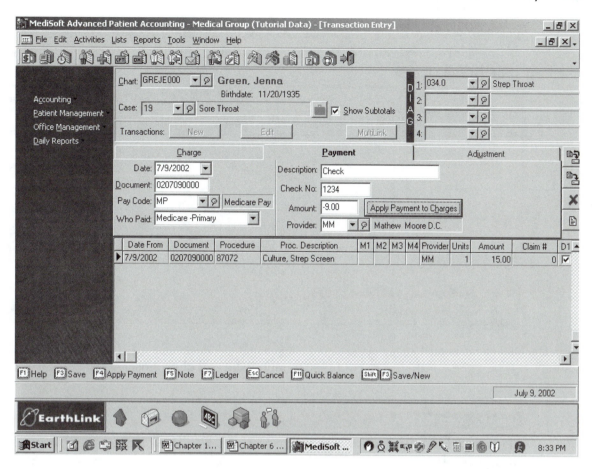

- Before you enter the adjustment, press apply payment to charges. Procedure charges and payments are linked through the apply payment to charges dialog box. A dialog box appears, where you can enter the payment.

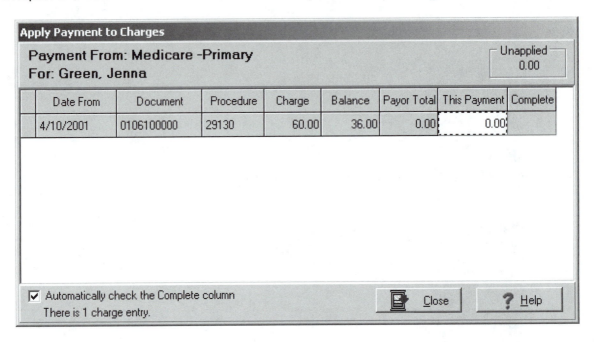

- Fill in the amount paid and click close.

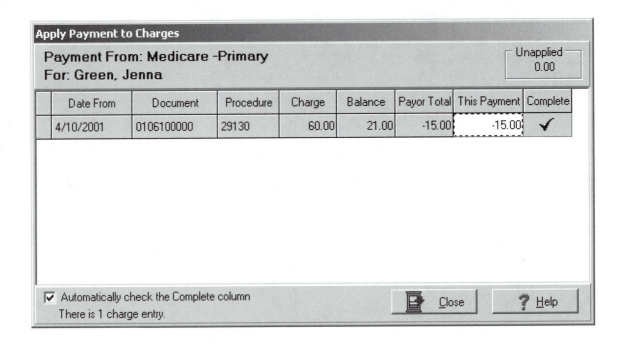

- Click on the adjustment tab.
- Fill in the amount of the adjustment (negative number) and the adjustment code (from a drop-down list).
- Click apply adjustment to charges and a dialog box appears in which you can enter and apply the adjustment.

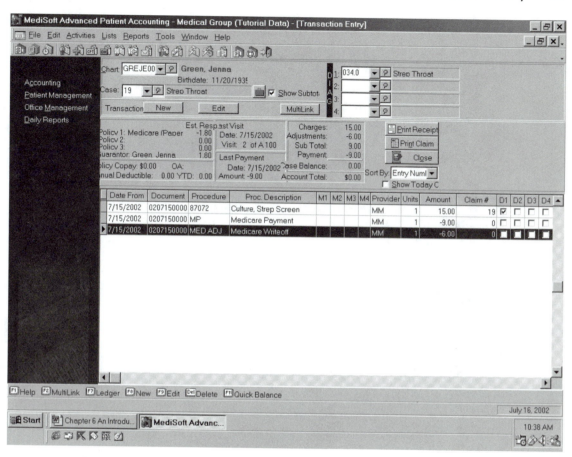

- You can now either edit the existing transaction or add a new one.
- To create a new transaction for Jenna's broken finger, click on the new command button and fill in the relevant information.
- Print the claim by clicking on the **print claim** button.

  After filling in all transactions for Jenna, you can see each of them on the transaction screen. Claims can also be created in the create claims dialog box.

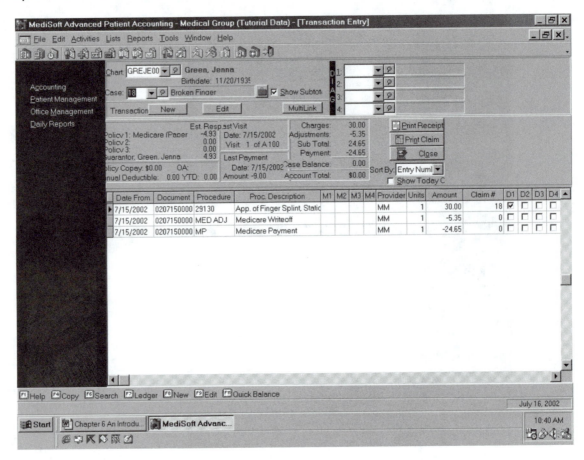

You can also see them listed in a **patient statement** by clicking reports, patient statements, and start; filling in Green's chart number for the beginning and end of the range; and printing.

CLAIM MANAGEMENT

You can see the billing status of your claims by printing a primary claim summary. Click on the reports menu and click custom report list. Select primary claim summary. Click OK. Click start. Fill in only the case numbers (18 and 19) and click OK.

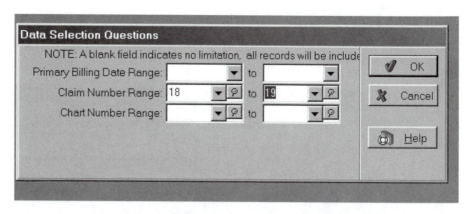

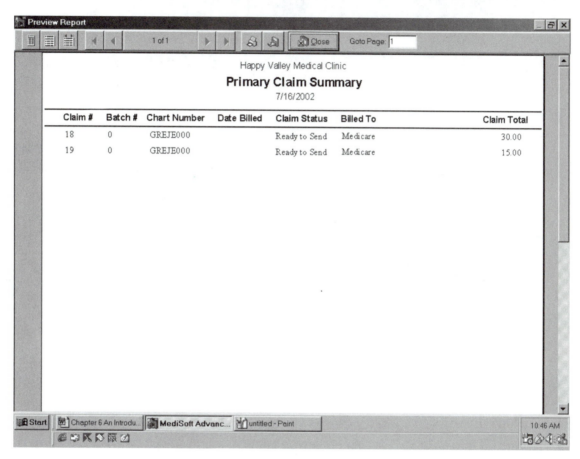

- Be sure to save each dialog box as you fill it in.

Printing a Primary Claim Summary   You may now print a primary claim summary for Jenna by doing the following:

- Pull down the reports menu and choose custom report list.
- Select primary claim summary.

- Click start.
- Fill in GREJE000 in both the chart number range dialog boxes.

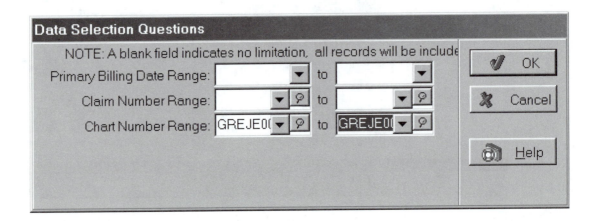

- Click OK.
- You can see the status of the claim and print it.

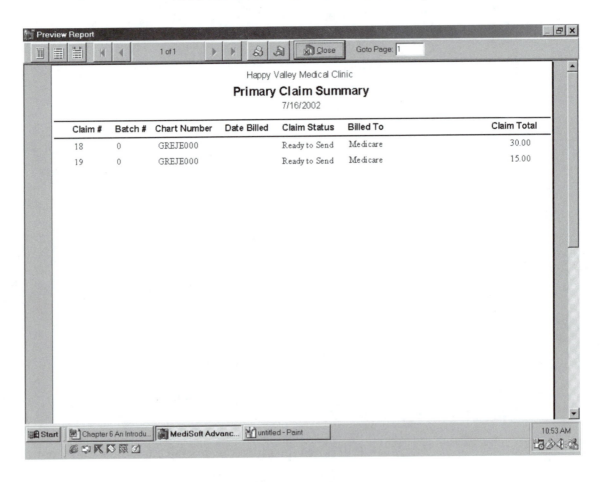

On this list, both claims are ready to send.

To add a new claim for Tonya Brown, do the following:

- Pull down the activities menu and select enter transactions.
- Enter the chart number of the patient BROTA000.

To enter a new transaction for Tonya Brown, do the following:

- Pull down the activities menu and select enter transactions. The following dialog box will appear:

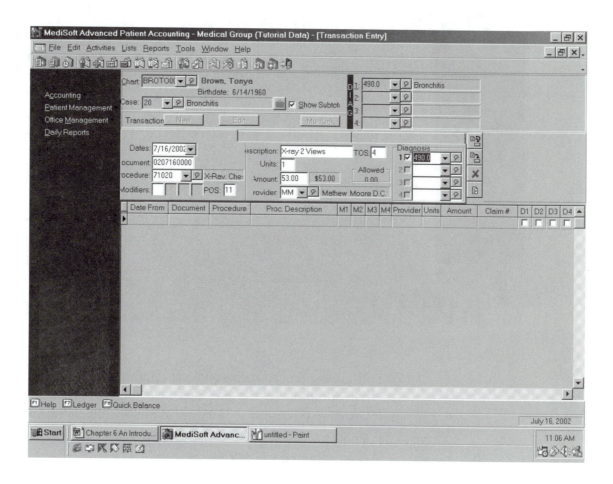

- Fill in the chart number and press enter; MediSoft fills in the rest of the information.
- Click on the print claim command button.

- Click the new command button, and the following dialog box will appear:

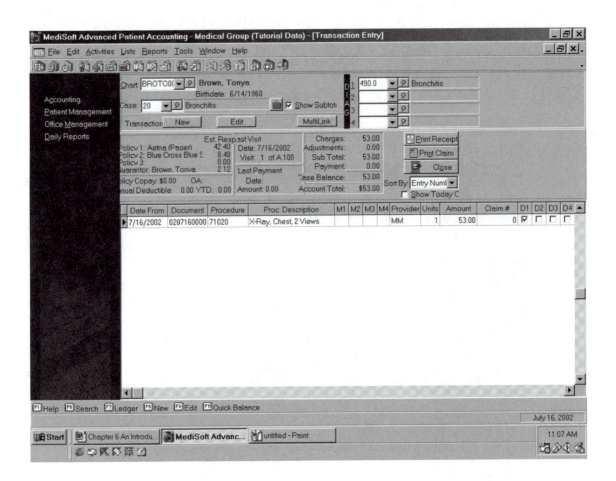

- Fill in the procedure by clicking on the down-arrow in the procedure drop-down list box and selecting X-ray chest, 2 views. Once the procedure is filled in, MediSoft fills in the charge.

- You also need to fill in the description of the payment. In this case, enter the word "check."

- Click print claim by clicking the print icon on the right.

- Click the new command button.

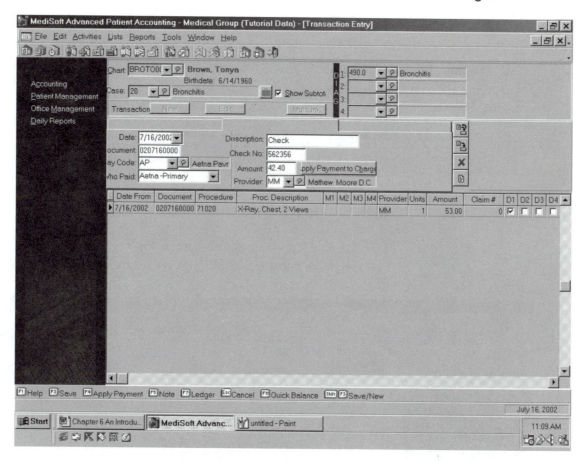

- Save the transaction.
- Click apply payment to charges, and the following dialog box will appear:

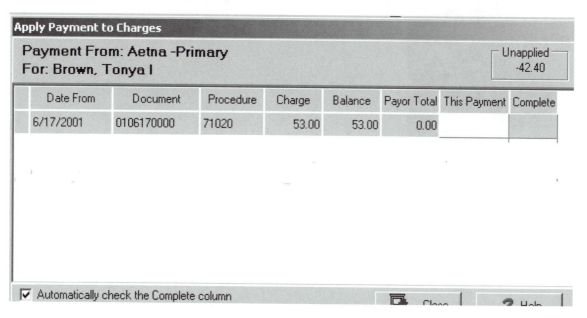

• Fill in 42.40 as the payment.

	Date From	Document	Procedure	Charge	Balance	Payor Total	This Payment	Complete
	6/17/2001	0106170000	71020	53.00	10.60	-42.40	-42.40	✓

Apply Payment to Charges

Payment From: Aetna -Primary
For: Brown, Tonya I

Unapplied
0.00

MediSoft applies the payment and closes the account.

• Look at the Transaction screen for Tonya. You can see that her secondary insurer (BC/BS) has paid the balance of $8.48.

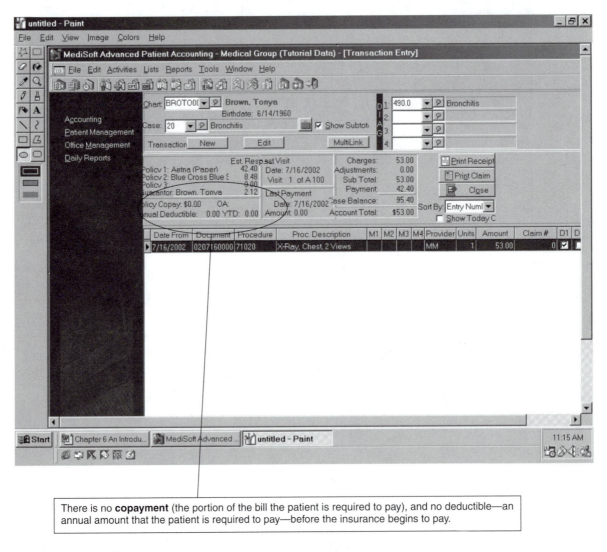

There is no **copayment** (the portion of the bill the patient is required to pay), and no deductible—an annual amount that the patient is required to pay—before the insurance begins to pay.

Because there are no adjustments, click save and close the window. The patient is billed for the remainder after the check and EOB (explanation of benefits) are received from BC/BS.

On your own, enter a transaction for yourself by pulling down the activities menu and entering your own chart number.

- Fill in the required information and click new.
- Click apply payment to charges.
- Fill in the payment (55.00) and close the dialog box. Be sure to save. You can see that the HMO (Cigna) paid the whole bill.
- Print the **patient face sheet**.

Because Kathy Patel has no insurance, a claim does not have to be generated for her. She is handed a bill at the end of a visit, and pays it. After paying, Kathy is handed a walkout receipt.

To see the status of all of your office's insurance claims, pull down the activities menu and select claim management.

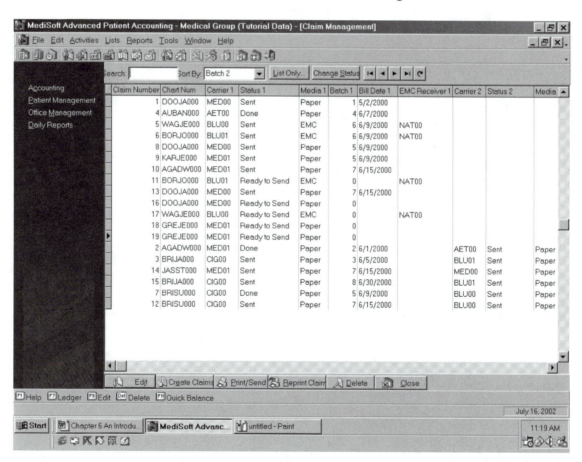

The screen shows the status of every claim. The claims are organized in **batches**, according to when they were created. The status of a claim includes whether it was submitted on paper or electronically, whether it is ready to send or has been sent to the primary insurer, the response from the primary insurer, whether or not claims are ready to send or have been sent to the secondary carrier. The status of each claim includes the response from the carrier. Each task has a date associated with it.

We have been creating claims from the transaction entry window; however, you can create claims another way—by clicking on the create claims command button at the bottom of the Deposits and Payments window.

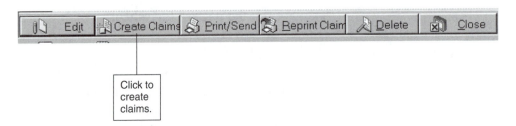

Click to create claims.

Claims can also be printed and sent, reprinted, or deleted using these command buttons.

ENTERING DEPOSITS

Payments must be deposited. They are automatically listed on the **deposit list** when you apply a payment. Enter a new transaction by doing the following:

- Pull down the activities menu.
- Choose deposits and payments. The following list appears:

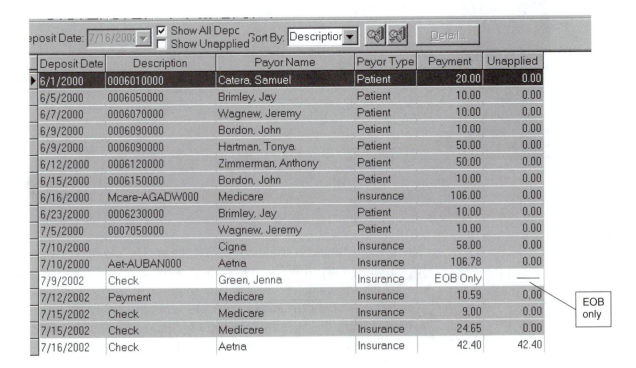

Deposit Date	Description	Payor Name	Payor Type	Payment	Unapplied
6/1/2000	0006010000	Catera, Samuel	Patient	20.00	0.00
6/5/2000	0006050000	Brimley, Jay	Patient	10.00	0.00
6/7/2000	0006070000	Wagnew, Jeremy	Patient	10.00	0.00
6/9/2000	0006090000	Bordon, John	Patient	10.00	0.00
6/9/2000	0006090000	Hartman, Tonya	Patient	50.00	0.00
6/12/2000	0006120000	Zimmerman, Anthony	Patient	50.00	0.00
6/15/2000	0006150000	Bordon, John	Patient	10.00	0.00
6/16/2000	Mcare-AGADW000	Medicare	Insurance	106.00	0.00
6/23/2000	0006230000	Brimley, Jay	Patient	10.00	0.00
7/5/2000	0007050000	Wagnew, Jeremy	Patient	10.00	0.00
7/10/2000		Cigna	Insurance	58.00	0.00
7/10/2000	Aet-AUBAN000	Aetna	Insurance	106.78	0.00
7/9/2002	Check	Green, Jenna	Insurance	EOB Only	—
7/12/2002	Payment	Medicare	Insurance	10.59	0.00
7/15/2002	Check	Medicare	Insurance	9.00	0.00
7/15/2002	Check	Medicare	Insurance	24.65	0.00
7/16/2002	Check	Aetna	Insurance	42.40	42.40

EOB only

• Note that the last transaction was an EOB only. The check was not applied. Payments can be applied when entering transactions or by pulling down the activities menu and choosing enter payments/deposits, clicking on the record, and clicking the apply command button.

The following dialog box appears.

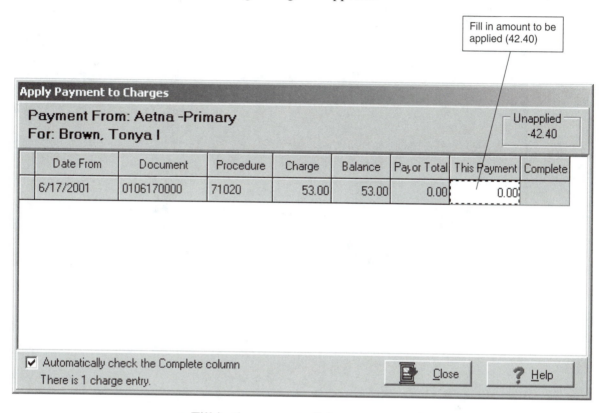

• Fill in the amount of the payment to be applied and close the dialog box.

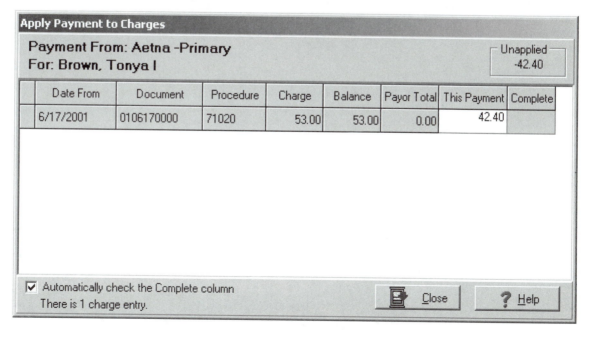

- The 42.40 will appear as applied in the deposit list.

Deposit Date: 7/16/200☐ ☑ Show All Depc ☐ Show Unapplied   Sort By: Descriptior ▾   [Detail...]

	Deposit Date	Description	Payor Name	Payor Type	Payment	Unapplied
	6/1/2000	0006010000	Catera, Samuel	Patient	20.00	0.00
	6/5/2000	0006050000	Brimley, Jay	Patient	10.00	0.00
	6/7/2000	0006070000	Wagnew, Jeremy	Patient	10.00	0.00
	6/9/2000	0006090000	Bordon, John	Patient	10.00	0.00
	6/9/2000	0006090000	Hartman, Tonya	Patient	50.00	0.00
	6/12/2000	0006120000	Zimmerman, Anthony	Patient	50.00	0.00
	6/15/2000	0006150000	Bordon, John	Patient	10.00	0.00
	6/16/2000	Mcare-AGADW000	Medicare	Insurance	106.00	0.00
	6/23/2000	0006230000	Brimley, Jay	Patient	10.00	0.00
	7/5/2000	0007050000	Wagnew, Jeremy	Patient	10.00	0.00
	7/10/2000		Cigna	Insurance	58.00	0.00
	7/10/2000	Aet-AUBAN000	Aetna	Insurance	106.78	0.00
	7/9/2002	Check	Green, Jenna	Insurance	EOB Only	——
	7/12/2002	Payment	Medicare	Insurance	10.59	0.00
	7/15/2002	Check	Medicare	Insurance	9.00	0.00
	7/15/2002	Check	Medicare	Insurance	24.65	0.00
▶	7/16/2002	Check	Aetna	Insurance	42.40	0.00

Check from Aetna

QUICK LEDGER AND QUICK BALANCE

If you want a quick summary of a patient's procedures or billing and payment status, pull down the activities menu and select quick ledger. Enter the chart number of the patient, and the following will appear:

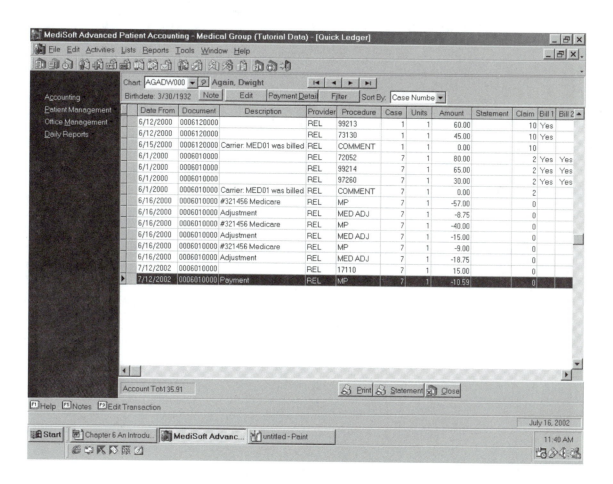

It can be printed by clicking on the print icon on the bottom of the screen.

If you simply want the patient's balance, pull down the activities menu and select quick balance. Enter the chart number of the patient, and the following will appear:

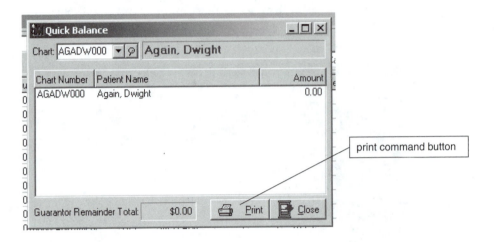

This can be printed by clicking on the print command button.

☐ NEW STYLE TRANSACTION ENTRY

Enter a new case for Dwight Again. On the personal tab of the case dialog box, enter the following:

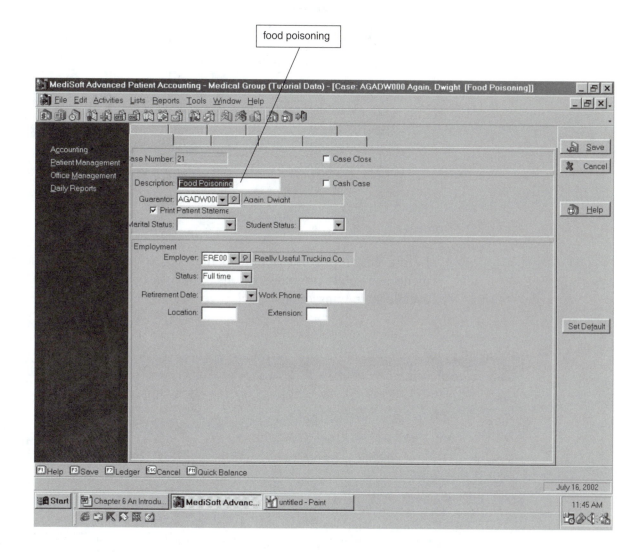

On the diagnosis tab, select the diagnosis (food poisoning) from the drop-down list box.

Click the condition tab and fill in the following:

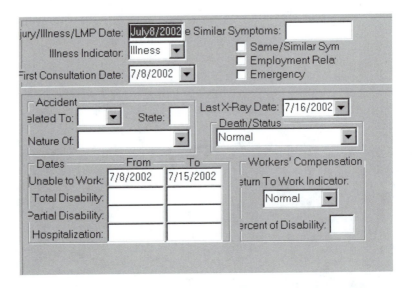

Before entering a transaction in the new style, pull down the file menu and select program options. Click on data entry and click off use old style transactions. Click save.

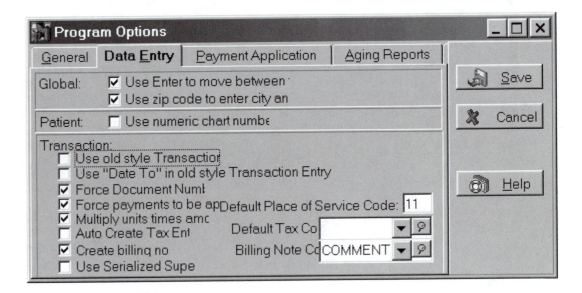

Click activities, and select enter transactions. The following window will be displayed:

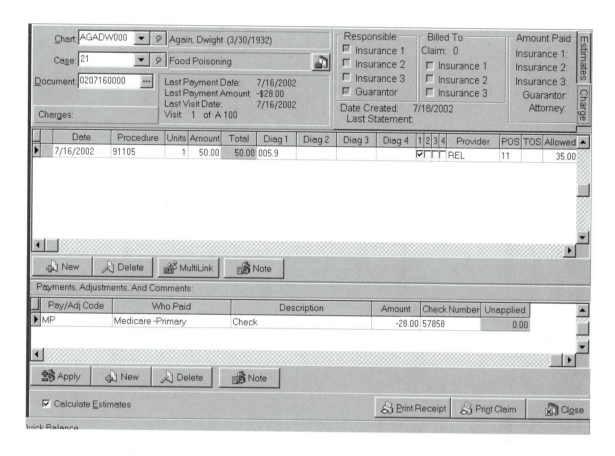

Make sure the charges tab on the extreme right side of the window is selected.

In new style transaction entry, you can enter procedure charges, payments, and apply payments in the same window. Click the new command button on the bottom of the top pane of the window to enter procedure charge information. Click new on the bottom of the lower window pane to enter payment transaction information. Click apply to apply the payment. This information will automatically be saved. You can also print receipts and create claims from this window.

Chapter Summary

- A transaction is a charge, payment, or adjustment to a patient account.
- A claim is a bill to an insurance carrier.
- Deposits are automatically entered on the deposit list when a payment is applied to a charge.

- The quick ledger shows you a quick summary of a patient's procedures and billing and payment status.
- The quick balance function shows a patient's balance.
- New style transaction entry allows the user to enter procedure charges, payments, and apply payments to charges in one window.

Key Words

Adjustment
Allowed amount
Assigned provider
Batches
Case number
Charges
Chart number
Copayment
Custom report

Deposit list
Patient face sheet
Patient statement
Payment
Primary claim summary
Procedure
Quick balance
Quick ledger
Walkout receipt

REVIEW EXERCISES

1. On your own, edit Jenna's transaction record to record a 24.65 payment from Medicare. Print the deposit report; the last entry should be a check from Medicare for 24.65. Start by pulling down the activities menu and selecting enter payments/deposits. Click apply. The following dialog box will appear:

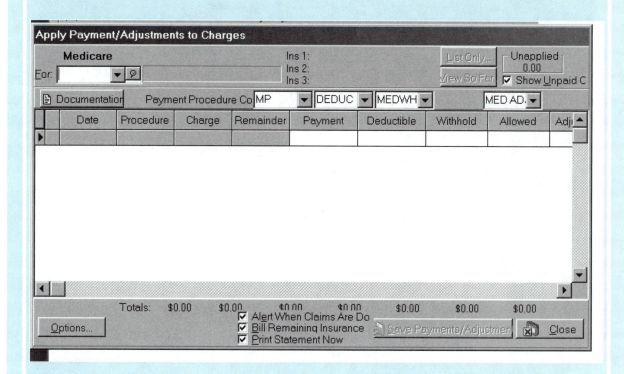

Click off show unpaid claims. Select Jenna's chart number. Fill in $24.65 as the payment and click save payments/adjustments. Close the dialog box and the applied payment should show on the deposit list.

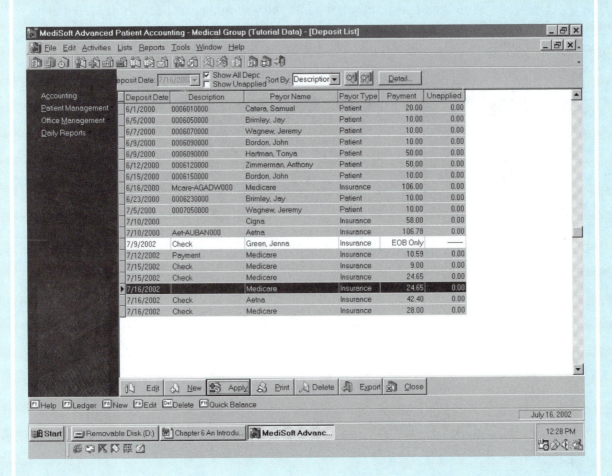

Chapter

7

Electronic Media Claims

Chapter Outline

- Learning Objectives
- Submitting Electronic Media Claims
- Electronic Claim Management
- Electronic Transfer of Funds
- Audit/Edit Report
- Chapter Summary
- Key Words
- Review Exercises

Learning Objectives

After completing this chapter, the student will

- Understand the process of submitting electronic claims
- Know what information must be in place before an electronic claim is submitted
- Understand the function of a clearinghouse
- Appreciate the differences between paper claims and electronic claims
- Understand the utilization of an audit/edit report

PLEASE NOTE THAT THIS CHAPTER IS FOR THE STUDENT'S IN-
FORMATION ONLY. THESE TASKS CANNOT BE PERFORMED IN A
CLASSROOM SETTING BECAUSE THE STUDENT DOES NOT HAVE
ACCESS TO A CLEARINGHOUSE OR ANY INSURANCE COMPANY.
THE ELECTRONIC CLAIM CAN ONLY BE SUBMITTED IN A REAL
HEALTH CARE OFFICE SETTING.

SUBMITTING ELECTRONIC MEDIA CLAIMS

Claims can be submitted to insurance carriers either on paper or electronically (EMC). The way this is done varies regionally. Some advantages are claimed for the electronic media claims (EMC) over the
paper claims. According to MediSoft (MediSoft Training Manual
Version 6.1, 5-3), the following is a comparison:

Compared Item	Electronic Claim	Paper Claim
Transactions Per Claim	13	6
Average Turnaround	7–14 Days	6–8 Weeks
Claim Tracking	Verification/Batch Numbers	None
Edits	Yes	No
Accuracy/Paid first time	98%	70%
Cost Per Claim	Free/$0.39	$0.35

A health care provider's office may choose to submit electronic
claims directly to an insurer or through a clearinghouse (a business
that collects claims from many offices and forwards them to the correct insurance carriers).

Several tasks must be completed by the user before electronic claims
can be submitted.

The information for patients, EMC receivers, insurance carriers,
providers, and referring providers must be entered. To access the following lists, pull down the lists menu and choose the appropriate option. Any of these lists can be edited or amended by the user.

MediSoft's tutorial includes a list of patients.

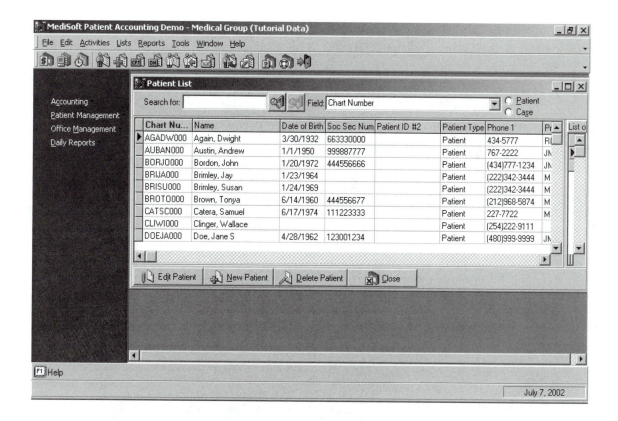

The tutorial database also has a table of EMC receivers set up.

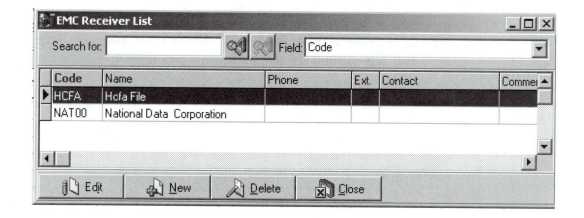

A list of insurance carriers is included as well.

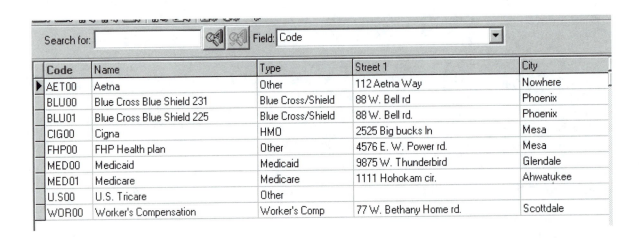

The tutorial database also contains a list of providers.

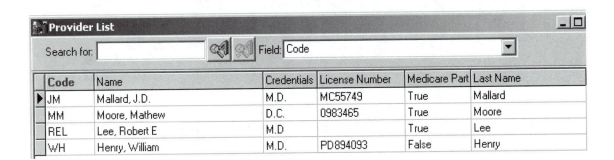

In addition, a referring provider list is included in the tutorial. The user can edit this list and add a new provider by clicking on the new command button near the bottom of the window. Fill in the following information:

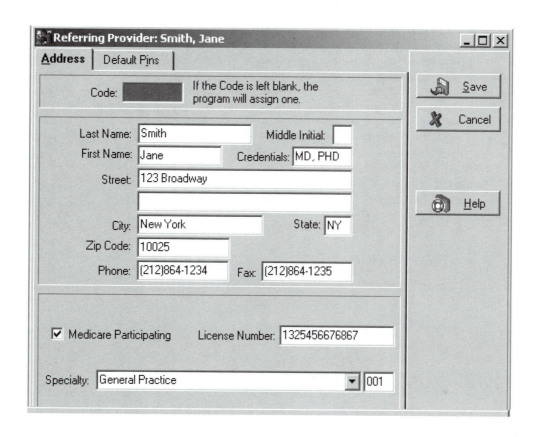

Click save and Jane Smith's name will appear on the provider list.

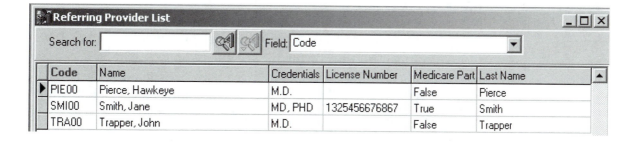

Although as a student you cannot create electronic claims, you can look at the claim management screen and see the various types of claim submissions. Pull down the activities menu and select claim management.

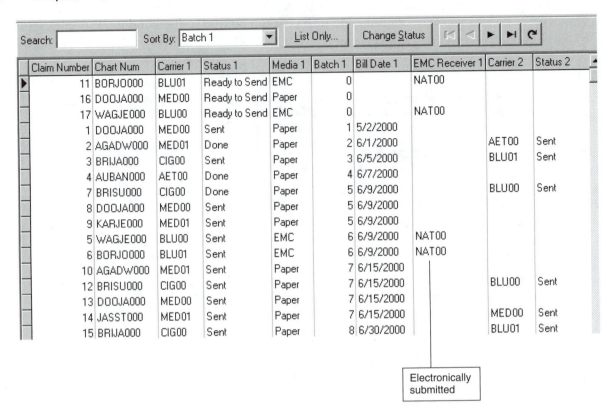

	Claim Number	Chart Num	Carrier 1	Status 1	Media 1	Batch 1	Bill Date 1	EMC Receiver 1	Carrier 2	Status 2
▶	11	BORJO000	BLU01	Ready to Send	EMC	0		NAT00		
	16	DOOJA000	MED00	Ready to Send	Paper	0				
	17	WAGJE000	BLU00	Ready to Send	EMC	0		NAT00		
	1	DOOJA000	MED00	Sent	Paper	1	5/2/2000			
	2	AGADW000	MED01	Done	Paper	2	6/1/2000		AET00	Sent
	3	BRIJA000	CIG00	Sent	Paper	3	6/5/2000		BLU01	Sent
	4	AUBAN000	AET00	Done	Paper	4	6/7/2000			
	7	BRISU000	CIG00	Done	Paper	5	6/9/2000		BLU00	Sent
	8	DOOJA000	MED00	Sent	Paper	5	6/9/2000			
	9	KARJE000	MED01	Sent	Paper	5	6/9/2000			
	5	WAGJE000	BLU00	Sent	EMC	6	6/9/2000	NAT00		
	6	BORJO000	BLU01	Sent	EMC	6	6/9/2000	NAT00		
	10	AGADW000	MED01	Sent	Paper	7	6/15/2000			
	12	BRISU000	CIG00	Sent	Paper	7	6/15/2000		BLU00	Sent
	13	DOOJA000	MED00	Sent	Paper	7	6/15/2000			
	14	JASST000	MED01	Sent	Paper	7	6/15/2000		MED00	Sent
	15	BRIJA000	CIG00	Sent	Paper	8	6/30/2000		BLU01	Sent

Electronically submitted

ELECTRONIC CLAIM MANAGEMENT

In order to submit claims electronically, you and the insurance carrier need a modem and a phone line. Many health care providers find it to be an expedient way of submitting claims. Electronic claims are considered more efficient and less expensive than paper submissions.

ELECTRONIC TRANSFER OF FUNDS

Electronic claims can be paid by electronic funds transfer (EFT), the electronic transfer of funds. The funds transfer can be accompanied by an electronic remittance advice (ERA), explaining the response to the claim. It is similar to the explanation of benefits (EOB) that accompanies the response to a paper claim.

Certain information is required for electronic claims to be submitted to Medicare. These include the patient's first and last names and signature on file in the Patient/Guarantor's dialog box, and the insured's policy and group number in the Case dialog box, Policy 1 tab. In the Transaction entry dialog box, Charge tab, dates and place of service, procedures, charges and units of service are also required. Provider information must include: signature on file, full name, PIN, and full adddress and phone. The practice information must include the Practice Name.

AUDIT/EDIT REPORT

If your office uses a clearinghouse to process electronic claims, it utilizes an audit/edit report to report whether all the necessary information is included and accurate.

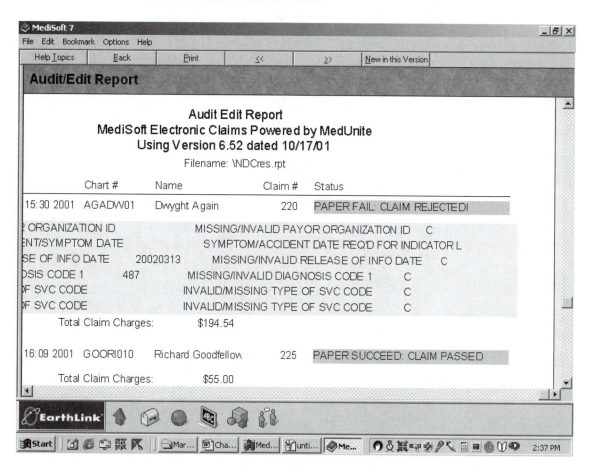

Chapter Summary

- Electronic media claims are submitted to insurance carriers via modem and phone line.
- Certain data (patients, EMC receivers, insurance carriers, providers, and referring providers) have to be in place before claims can be submitted electronically.
- Electronic funds transfer can be used to satisfy electronically submitted claims by transferring funds from one bank to another.
- An electronic remittance advice explains the insurance company's response.
- An audit/edit report can be used to check for errors.

Key Words

Audit/edit report
Electronic funds transfer (EFT)

Electronic remittance advice
(ERA)

REVIEW EXERCISES

Define the following terms:

1. Clearinghouse
2. Electronic media claim
3. Electronic remittance advice
4. Audit/edit report
5. Electronic funds transfer

Critical Thinking

1. Explain the advantages and disadvantages of using electronic claim management versus paper billing.

Chapter

8

Printing Reports

Chapter Outline

Learning Objectives

Upon completion of this chapter, the student will

- Be able to generate various kinds of reports whose structure is provided by MediSoft

- Be able to use a filter to select records to display in the reports
- Be aware of the uses of day sheets, aging reports, patient statements, patient ledger, analysis reports, and several others
- Appreciate the different uses of the many reports provided

INTRODUCTION

MediSoft provides structures for all types of reports. The user selects the report structure, and **filters** out records that he or she is not interested in by filling out a data selection screen specifying a range of chart numbers and dates. MediSoft then fills in the contents of the report—putting data from a file into the report structure chosen.

DAY SHEETS

Patient Day Sheets   MediSoft provides many reports which can present data in an attractive and useful format. A patient day sheet is used for daily reconciliation. It lists the day's transactions. To create a patient day sheet for Tonya Brown, select day sheets. From the fly-out menu, select patient day sheet. The following window is displayed. In the print report where? window, make sure preview the report on the screen is chosen and click start.

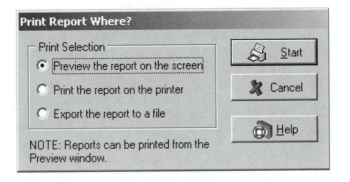

On the data selection screen, enter Tonya's chart number in both the from and to boxes. Delete the dates and then click OK.

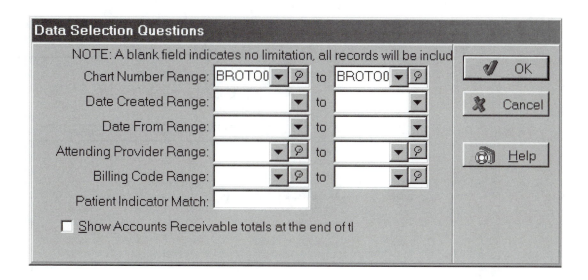

The following report will be generated:

Happy Valley Medical Clinic
Patient Day Sheet
Ending 7/16/2002

Entry	Date	Document	POS	Description	Provider	Code	Amount
BROTO000		Tonya Brown					
123	7/16/2002	0207160000	11	X-ray 2 Views	MM	71020	53.00
125	7/16/2002	0207160000		#562356 Aetna	MM	AP	-42.40
		Patient's Charges		Patient's Receipts	Adjustments		Patient Balance
		$53.00		-$42.40	$0.00		$10.60

Close the preview screen by clicking on the close command button toward the top of the window.

Procedure Day Sheets A patient day sheet lists procedures, codes, and amounts owed under each patient. On the other hand, a procedure day sheet lists a procedure and grouped under the procedure, along with how much money each service earned, are all the patients who underwent that procedure. To create a procedure day sheet choose reports, day sheets, procedure day sheet. Click start. In the data selection box, delete the dates, and do not add chart numbers. You will get a report listing every day, every patient, grouped under the procedure name. Click create. The following report will appear:

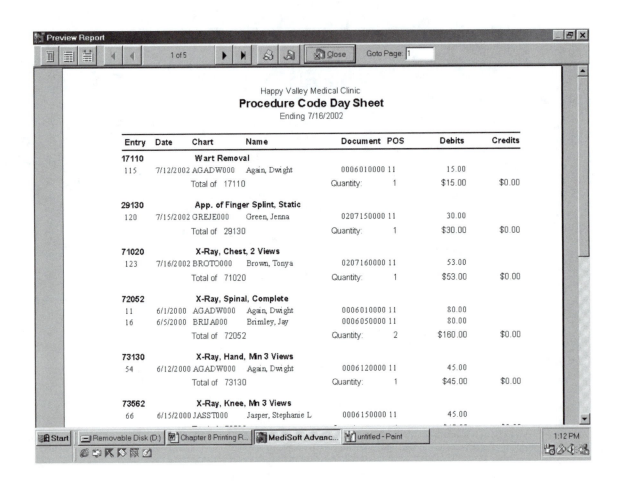

Close the preview screen by clicking on the close command button toward the top of the window.

Payment Day Sheets   Follow the same steps (leaving the data selection dialog box blank— no dates, no providers) to generate a payment day sheet. The payment day sheet groups patients under their health care providers, so that the user can see the payments received by each provider.

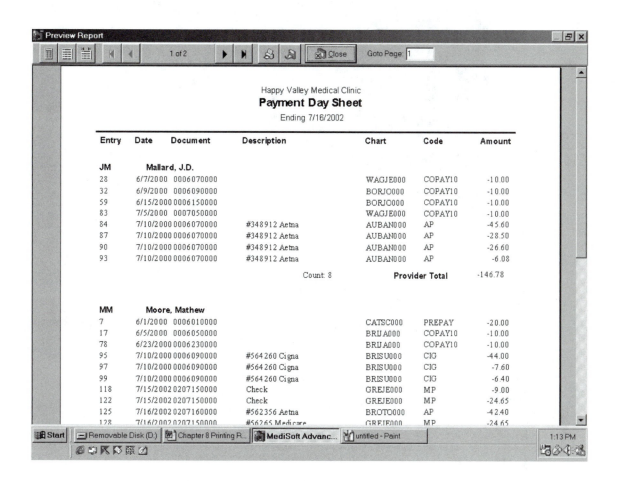

Close the preview screen by clicking on the close command button toward the top of the window.

BILLING/PAYMENT STATUS REPORT

To print a **billing/payment status report**, which shows current billing, payment, and claim status of each transaction, pull down the reports menu and select analysis reports.

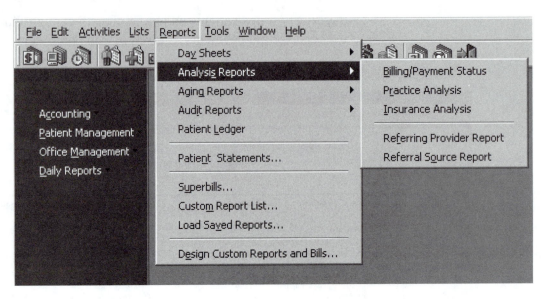

From the fly-out menu, select billing/payment status report. Click start. On the data selection screen, leave all boxes blank. Click OK, and the following report is generated.

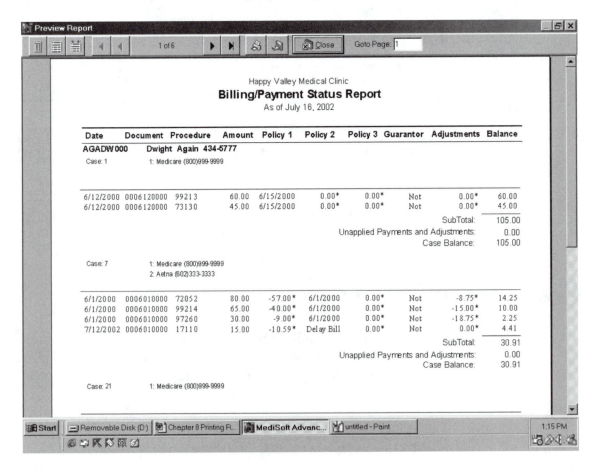

Close the preview screen by clicking on the close command button toward the top of the window.

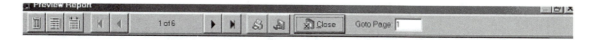

ANALYSIS REPORTS

Practice Analysis Reports   A practice analysis report is usually generated monthly. However, it can be used for any specified time, for example, quarter or year. It provides a summary of activity for the period chosen. Click start. Leave all fields on the data selection screen blank, and click OK. The following report is generated.

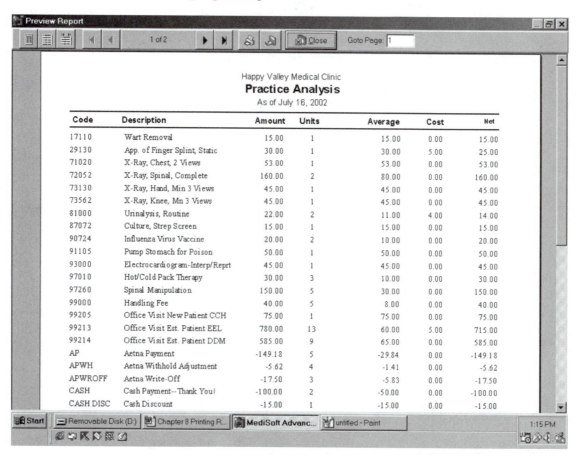

As you can see, all procedure codes and descriptions are listed, with the charge, the number of times the procedure was performed, the average charge, any costs, and the net. Close the preview screen by clicking on the close command button toward the top of the window.

Insurance Analysis Reports   An **insurance analysis report** is created by pulling down the reports menu, selecting analysis reports, and then insurance analysis report.

Click start. On the next screen, leave all data selection fields blank and click OK.

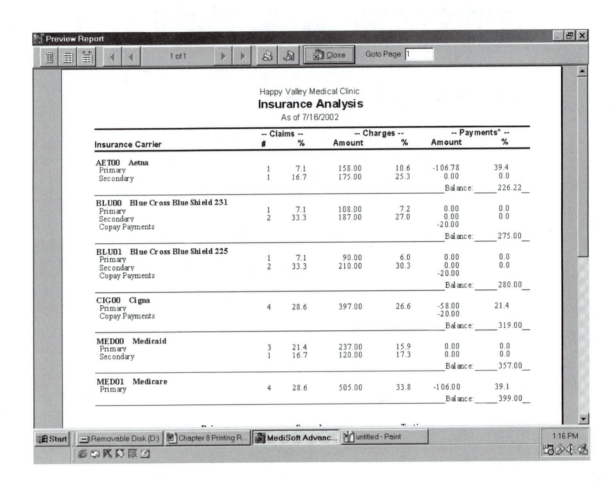

This report lists each insurance carrier that has been billed, amounts and percentages of claims, charges, and payments. Close the preview screen by clicking on the close command button toward the top of the window.

AGING REPORTS

Patient Aging Reports   To create a patient aging report, pull down the reports menu, choose aging reports, and select patient aging. Click start. Leave all data selection questions blank and click OK.

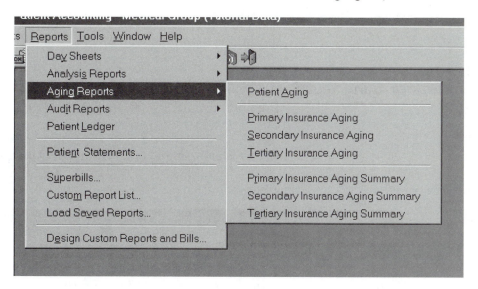

A patient aging report lists the patient with the amounts owed to the practice by age (current 0–30, past due 31–60, past due 61–90, and over 90). It also lists the total amount each patient owes and each patient's phone number.

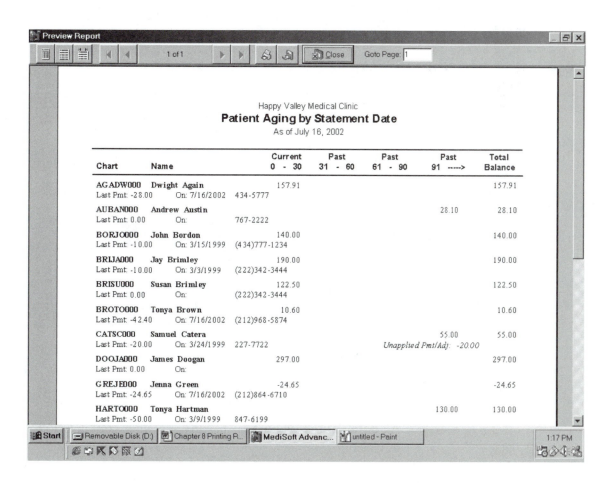

Close the preview screen by clicking on the close command button toward the top of the window.

Insurance Aging Report

An **insurance aging report** lists claims filed by age (current 0–30 from billing date, 31–60, 61–90, 91–999).

Below is an example of an Insurance Aging Report:

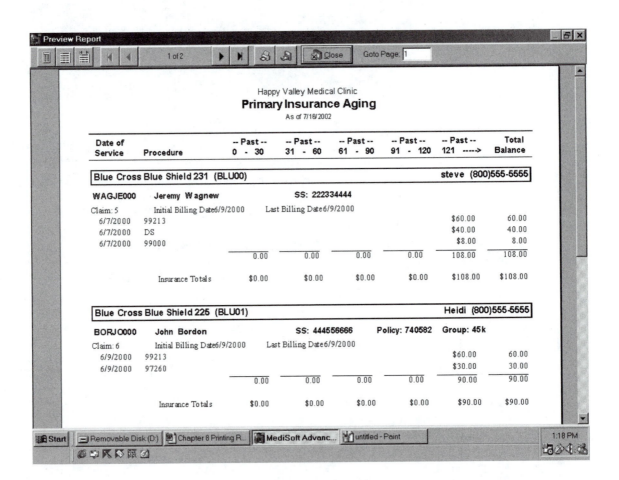

Close the preview screen by clicking on the close command button toward the top of the window.

DATA AUDIT REPORT

A **data audit report** lists any changes or deletions made in transactions.

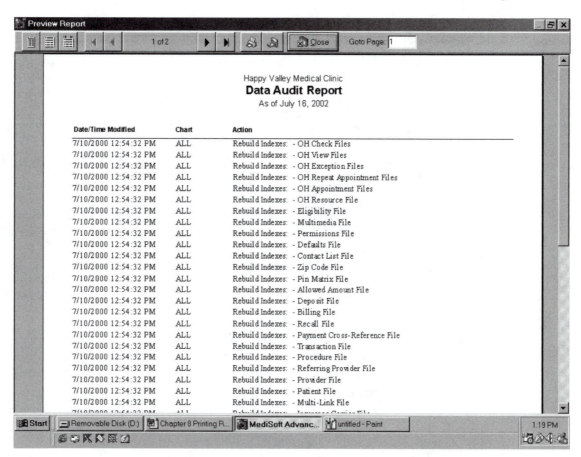

Close the preview screen by clicking on the close command button toward the top of the window.

PATIENT LEDGER

A **patient ledger** displays the status of each patient's account, past activity, and billing history. To print a patient ledger, pull down the reports menu and choose patient ledger, click start, and on the data selection window fill in as follows and click OK.

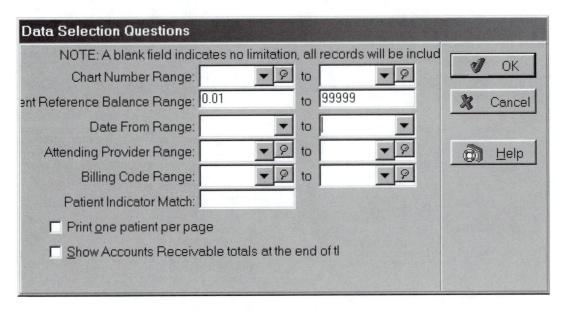

The following patient account ledger groups the information under each patient's chart number, name and date, and amount of last payment, place of service, description of the payment, procedure code, provider, and amount, with a total amount for each patient.

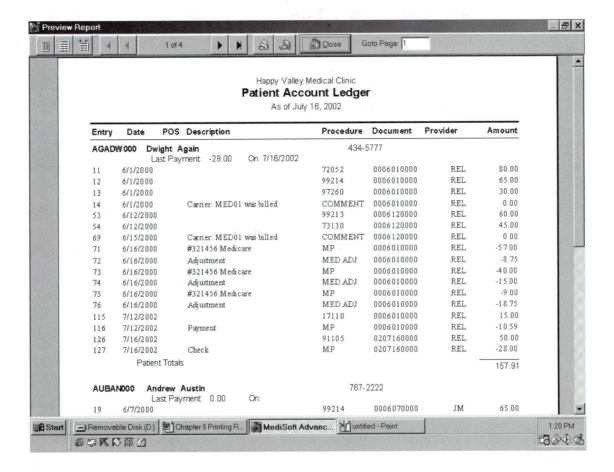

Close the preview screen by clicking on the close command button toward the top of the window.

PATIENT STATEMENTS

MediSoft provides several different statement formats. Like other reports, the patient statement can be filtered by selecting a particular date range and a particular patient or patients. To print a patient statement, click reports, then patient statements. The following dialog box is displayed:

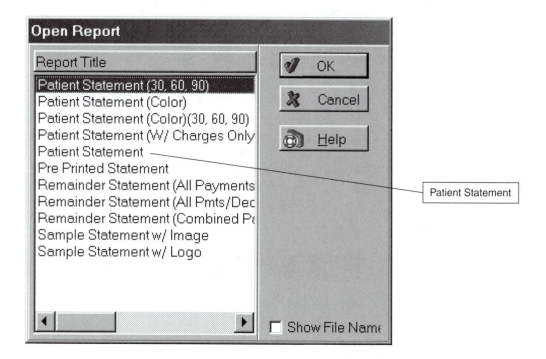

Choose patient statement, click start, and fill in the data selection dialog box as follows to filter out all patients except Tonya Brown. To print Tonya Brown's statement:

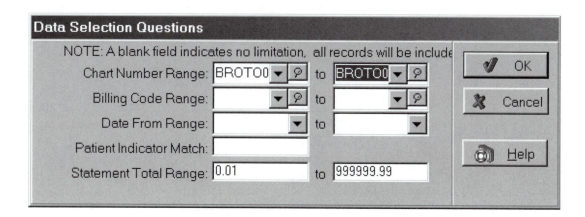

Click OK. The following statement appears on the screen and can be printed.

Happy Valley Medical Clinic
916 E. Baseline rd.
Mesa, AZ 85204
(800)333-4747

Statement Date	Page
7/16/2002	1

Tonya Brown
229 West 109th Street
New York, N 10025

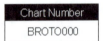

Chart Number
BROTO000

Date	Document	Description	Case Number	Amount
Date of Last Payment: 7/16/2002		Amount: -42.40	Previous Balance:	0.00
Patient: Tonya Brown		Chart #: BROTO000	Case Description: Bronchitis	
7/16/2002	0207160000	X-Ray, Chest, 2 Views	20	53.00
7/16/2002	0207160000	Aetna Payment	20	-42.40

Total Charges	Total Payments	Total Adjustments	Balance Due
$53.00	-$42.40	$0.00	**10.60**

As you can see, transactions for Tonya and her last payment are listed. Close the preview screen by clicking on the close command button toward the top of the window. The two addresses at the top allow you to send these statements in window envelopes.

REMAINDER STATEMENTS

A **remainder statement** is sent only after all insurance carriers have paid. If the complete box is checked, the remainder of the balance due is the responsibility of the guarantor. To generate a remainder statement, pull down the reports menu, choose patient statements and choose remainder statement (all payments).

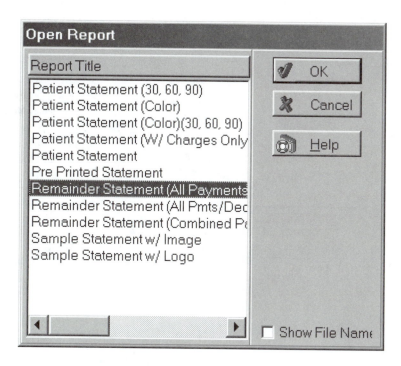

Click OK. Start. Fill in the data selection dialog box as follows for Dwight Again's remainder statement:

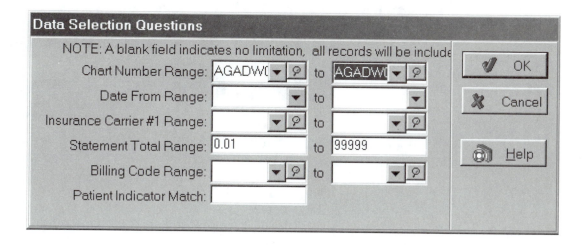

Click OK, and the following report will appear listing a patient's date of procedure, the procedure, the amounts paid by the primary and secondary insurers, and the remainder to be billed to the guarantor. Close the preview screen by clicking on the close command button toward the top of the window.

Happy Valley Medical Clinic
916 E. Baseline rd.
Suite 225
Mesa, AZ 85204
(800)333-4747

Dwight Again
1742 N. 83rd Ave.
Phoenix, AZ 85021

Statement Date	Chart Number	Page
07/16/2002	AGADW000	1

Make Checks Payable To:
Happy Valley Medical Clinic
916 E. Baseline rd.
Suite 225
Mesa, AZ 85204
(800)333-4747

Date of Last Payment: 7/16/2002 Amount: -28.00			Previous Balance: 0.00	
Patient: Dwight Again	Chart Number: AGADW000		Case: Food Poisoning	

Dates	Procedure	Charge	Paid by Primary	Paid By Guarantor	Adjustments	Remainder
07/16/02	91105	50.00	-28.00		0.00	22.00

Benefits will be paid to the Insured. Guarantor is responsible for balance.

CUSTOM REPORTS

MediSoft has many custom reports. Click on custom report list and the following list is displayed:

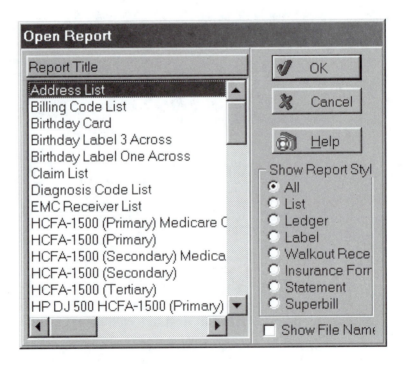

To see the rest of the custom reports, scroll down. Choose HCFA-1500 (primary) with form. Click start. Leave the data selection dialog box blank, and click OK. The filled-out HCFA form will appear on the screen.

PLEASE DO NOT STAPLE IN THIS AREA P		MEDICARE 1111 HOHOKAM CIR. AHWATUKEE, AZ 85678	

HEALTH INSURANCE CLAIM FORM

PICA						PICA

1. MEDICARE MEDICAID CHAMPUS CHAMPVA GROUP HEALTH PLAN FECA BLK LUNG OTHER	1a. INSURED'S I.D. NUMBER (FOR PROGRAM IN ITEM 1)
(Medicare #) (Medicaid #) (Sponsor's SSN) (VA File #) (SSN OR ID) (SSN or ID) (ID)	

2. PATIENT'S NAME (Last Name, First Name, Middle Initial) GREEN, JENNA	3. PATIENT'S BIRTH DATE SEX MM DD YY 11 20 35 M ☐ F ☒	4. INSURED'S NAME (Last Name, First Name, Middle Initial) GREEN, JENNA
5. PATIENT'S ADDRESS (No., Street) 6060 AMSTERDAM AVENUE	6. PATIENT RELATIONSHIP TO INSURED Self ☒ Spouse ☐ Child ☐ Other ☐	7. INSURED'S ADDRESS (No., Street) 6060 AMSTERDAM AVENUE
CITY NEW YORK STATE N	8. PATIENT STATUS Single ☐ Married ☐ Other ☐	CITY NEW YORK STATE N
ZIP CODE 10025 TELEPHONE (Include Area Code) (212) 864 6710	Employed ☐ Full-Time Student ☐ Part-Time Student ☐	ZIP CODE 10025 TELEPHONE (INCLUDE AREA CODE) (212) 864 6710

9. OTHER INSURED'S NAME (Last Name, First Name, Middle Initial)	10. IS PATIENT CONDITION RELATED TO:	11. INSURED'S POLICY GROUP OR FECA NUMBER
a. OTHER INSURED'S POLICY OR GROUP NUMBER	a. EMPLOYMENT? (CURRENT OR PREVIOUS) ☐ YES ☒ NO	a. INSURED'S DATE OF BIRTH SEX MM DD YY 11 20 35 M ☐ F ☒
b. OTHER INSURED'S DATE OF BIRTH SEX MM DD YY M ☐ F ☐	b. AUTO ACCIDENT? PLACE (State) ☐ YES ☒ NO	b. EMPLOYER'S NAME OR SCHOOL NAME
c. EMPLOYER'S NAME OR SCHOOL NAME	c. OTHER ACCIDENT? ☐ YES ☒ NO	c. INSURANCE PLAN NAME OR PROGRAM NAME
d. INSURANCE PLAN NAME OR PROGRAM NAME	10d. RESERVED FOR LOCAL USE	d. IS THERE ANOTHER HEALTH BENEFIT PLAN? ☐ YES ☒ NO If yes, return to and complete item 9a-d.

READ BACK OF FORM BEFORE COMPLETING AND SIGNING THIS FORM.

12. PATIENT'S OR AUTHORIZED PERSON'S SIGNATURE. I authorize the release of any medical or other information necessary to process this claim. I also request payment of government benefits either to myself or to the party who accepts assignment below. SIGNED _____ DATE _____	13. INSURED'S OR AUTHORIZED PERSON'S SIGNATURE. I authorize payment of medical benefits to the undersigned physician or supplier for services described below. SIGNED _____

14. DATE OF CURRENT: ILLNESS (First symptom) OR INJURY (Accident) OR PREGNANCY(LMP) MM DD YY	15. IF PATIENT HAS HAD SAME OR SIMILAR ILLNESS GIVE FIRST DATE MM DD YY	16. DATES PATIENT UNABLE TO WORK IN CURRENT OCCUPATION MM DD YY MM DD YY FROM _____ TO _____
17. NAME OF REFERRING PHYSICIAN OR OTHER SOURCE	17a. I.D. NUMBER OR REFERRING PHYSICIAN	18. HOSPITALIZATION DATES RELATED TO CURRENT SERVICES MM DD YY MM DD YY FROM _____ TO _____
19. RESERVED FOR LOCAL USE		20. OUTSIDE LAB? $ CHARGES ☐ YES ☒ NO

21. DIAGNOSIS OR NATURE OF ILLNESS OR INJURY (RELATE ITEMS 1,2,3 OR 4 TO ITEM 24 BY LINE)	22. MEDICAID RESUBMISSION CODE ORIGINAL REF. NO.
1. 034.0 ___ 3. ___ . ___	
2. ___ . ___ 4. ___ . ___	23. PRIOR AUTHORIZATION NUMBER

24. A DATE(S) OF SERVICE From To MM DD YY MM DD YY	B Place of Service	C Type of Service	D PROCEDURES, SERVICES, OR SUPPLIES (Explain unusual Circumstances) CPT/HCPCS	MODIFIER	E DIAGNOSIS CODE	F $ CHARGES	G DAY'S OR UNITS	H EPSDT Family Plan	I EMG	J COB	K RESERVED FOR LOCAL USE
07 15 02 07 15 02	11	5	87072		1	15.00	1				

Close the preview screen.

To look at superbills, choose superbill from the custom report list. Click start. Leave the data selection dialog box blank and click OK. It takes a little time to generate because it is hundreds of pages long. The first page looks like this:

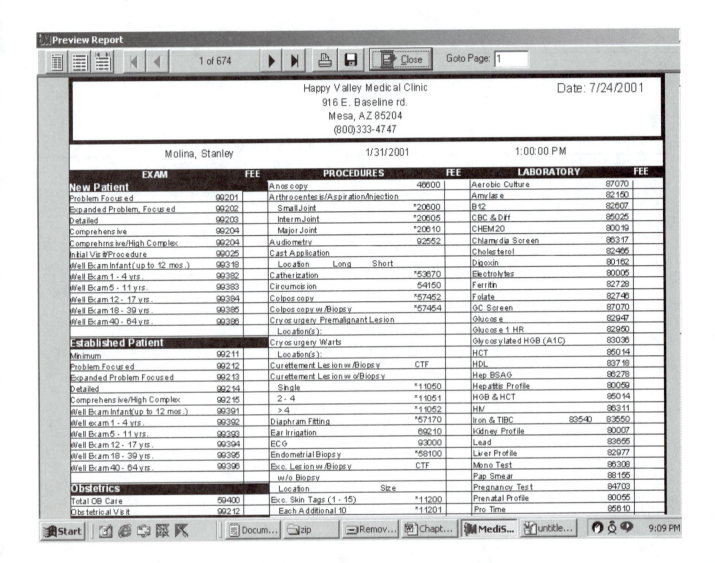

Close the preview screen by clicking on the close command button toward the top of the window.

A **walkout receipt** is given to the patient when he or she pays. It includes procedures performed and accounting codes. To print a walkout receipt, choose walkout receipt (all transactions) from the custom report list. Click start. Click OK. The following report is generated.

Happy Valley Medical Clinic
916 E. Baseline rd.
Mesa, AZ 85204
(800)333-4747

Page: 1

7/16/2002

Patient: Dwight Again
1742 N. 83rd Ave.
Phoenix, AZ 85021

Chart #: AGADW000
Case #: 1

Instructions:
Complete the patient information portion of your insurance claim form. Attach this bill, signed and dated, and all other bills pertaining to the claim. If you have a deductible policy, hold your claim forms until you have met your deductible. Mail directly to your insurance carrier.

Date	Description	Procedure	Modify	Dx 1	Dx 2	Dx 3	Dx 4	Units	Charge
6/12/2000	Office Visit Est. Patient EEL	99213		959.4				1	60.00
6/12/2000	X-Ray, Hand, Min 3 Views	73130		959.4				1	45.00
6/15/2000	COMMENT	COMMENT						1	0.00
6/12/2000	Office Visit Est. Patient EEL	99213		959.4				1	60.00
6/12/2000	X-Ray, Hand, Min 3 Views	73130		959.4				1	45.00
6/15/2000	COMMENT	COMMENT						1	0.00
6/12/2000	Office Visit Est. Patient EEL	99213		959.4				1	60.00
6/12/2000	X-Ray, Hand, Min 3 Views	73130		959.4				1	45.00
6/15/2000	COMMENT	COMMENT						1	0.00
6/12/2000	Office Visit Est. Patient EEL	A2000		959.4				1	60.00
6/15/2000	COMMENT	COMMENT		959.4				1	0.00
6/12/2000	Office Visit Est. Patient EEL	99213		959.4				1	60.00
6/12/2000	X-Ray, Hand, Min 3 Views	73130		959.4				1	45.00
6/15/2000	COMMENT	COMMENT						1	0.00
6/12/2000	Office Visit Est. Patient EEL	99213		959.4				1	60.00
6/12/2000	X-Ray, Hand, Min 3 Views	73130		959.4				1	45.00
6/15/2000	COMMENT	COMMENT						1	0.00
6/12/2000	Office Visit Est. Patient EEL	99213		959.4				1	60.00
6/12/2000	X-Ray, Hand, Min 3 Views	73130		959.4				1	45.00
6/15/2000	COMMENT	COMMENT						1	0.00
6/12/2000	Office Visit Est. Patient EEL	A2000		959.4				1	60.00
6/12/2000	X-Ray, Hand, Min 3 Views	73130		959.4				1	45.00
6/15/2000	COMMENT	COMMENT						1	0.00
6/12/2000	Office Visit Est. Patient EEL	99213		959.4				1	60.00
6/12/2000	X-Ray, Hand, Min 3 Views	73130		959.4				1	45.00
6/15/2000	COMMENT	COMMENT						1	0.00

Provider Information

Provider Name:	J.D. Mallard M.D.
License:	MC55749
Medicaid PIN:	222222
SSN or EIN:	FedtaxID

Total Charges:	$ 945.00
Total Payments:	$ 0.00
Total Adjustments:	$ 0.00
Total Due This Visit:	**$ 945.00**
Total Account Balance:	$ 0.00

Assign and Release: I hereby authorize payment of medical benefits to this physician for the services described above. I also authorize the release of any information necessary to process this claim.

Close the preview window by clicking on the close command button at the top of the window.

Chapter Summary

- MediSoft provides ready-made report structures for many kinds of statements, bills, lists, and reports.
- A patient day sheet lists the patient and under the patient the procedures, place of service, provider, amount, and total balance.
- A procedure day sheet lists a procedure and all the patients who underwent that procedure, including debits and credits.
- A payment day sheet lists the provider, and under the provider all procedures performed and the amount.
- A billing/payment status report presents a patient's billing status.
- A practice analysis report is generated periodically and lists procedures, charges, number of times the procedure was performed, the average charge for the procedure, costs to the practice, and the net.
- An insurance analysis report lists insurance carriers the practice submits claims to, the amounts claimed, and percent covered, charges, and payments. Each insurance carrier is listed as a primary and secondary. Required copayments are also included.
- Patient aging reports list amounts due and the number of days overdue.
- Insurance aging reports list amounts due on claims and the number of days overdue.
- A data audit report lists any changes in transactions.
- A patient ledger lists a patient's chart number, name, the amount and date of latest payment, provider, procedure code and amount, as well as summary totals for each patient.
- A patient statement lists a patient's procedures, case, and all payments received, including a balance.
- A remainder statement is a bill to the guarantor after all insurance is exhausted.
- HCFA-1500 is one of the many custom reports. It can be printed on the HCFA form. Superbills and walkout receipts are also custom reports.

Key Words

Billing/payment status report	Patient day sheet
Data audit report	Patient ledger
Filter	Remainder statement
Insurance aging report	Walkout receipt
Insurance analysis report	

REVIEW EXERCISES

Hands-on Exercises

1. Create a patient statement (30, 60, 90) for yourself. Pull down the reports menu, and choose patient statement (30, 60, 90). Click start. Fill in your chart number as from and to. (If you do not recall your chart number, enter the first three letters of your last name, and MediSoft will bring up your Chart Number.) Click OK. Print the statement and hand it in.

2. Create a patient aging statement for yourself. Print the statement and hand it in.

Matching Questions

Match the definition with the term.

_____Patient Aging Report

_____Remainder Statement

_____Billing/Payment Status Report

_____Patient Day Sheet

_____Data Audit Report

1. Report that indicates any changes and/or deletions made in the database.

2. Report that lists the amounts owed by a patient by how many days late the payment is.

3. Report that shows the status of all transactions that have a responsible carrier, showing who has paid and who has not been billed.

4. Report listing the day's transactions that is used for daily reconciliation.

5. Report that includes only procedures for which payment has been received or rejected by all applicable insurance carriers. The guarantor is responsible for the remainder.

Designing Reports

Chapter Outline

- Learning Objectives
- Designing Reports
- Creating a List
- Creating a Labels Report
- Creating a Custom Ledger Report
- Chapter Summary
- Key Words
- Review Exercises

Learning Objectives

Upon completion of this chapter, the student will

- Be aware of the many custom bills and reports MediSoft allows the user to design
- Know how to use the custom design grid to design several types of reports

DESIGNING REPORTS

If none of the reports MediSoft provides is useful to you, you can design your own. MediSoft provides a grid on which you may design the structure of a report. The user indicates what table the report should take the data from, as well as its placement. We use two data types: text, which does not change in the report (a report header is a report header), and data fields whose contents do change from **detail line** to detail line, because the report takes the actual data from a table that is already entered.

To design a simple report listing patient, chart number, and provider in list form, do the following:

- Click on reports, design custom reports and bills. You will see MediSoft's **report designer** with its own toolbar.

The Report Designer Toolbar

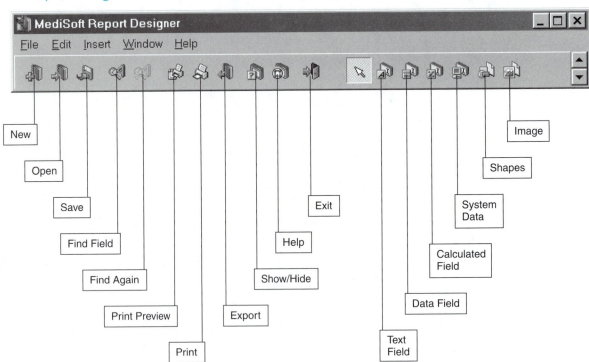

CREATING A LIST

To create a report in list style, do the following:

- Pull down the File menu and choose new. The following dialog box opens:

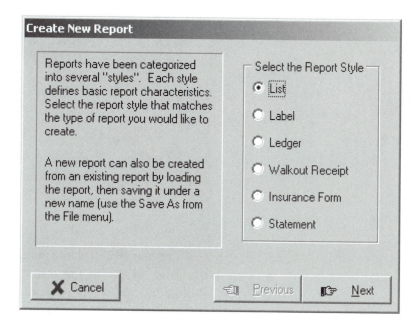

- Select list and click next. The following window is displayed:

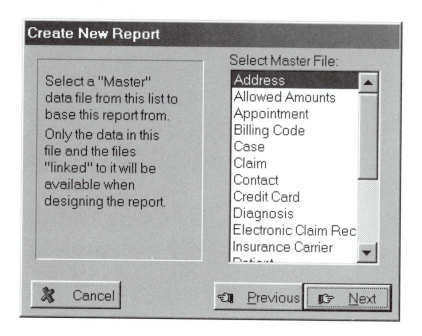

- Choose patient as the master file and click next.

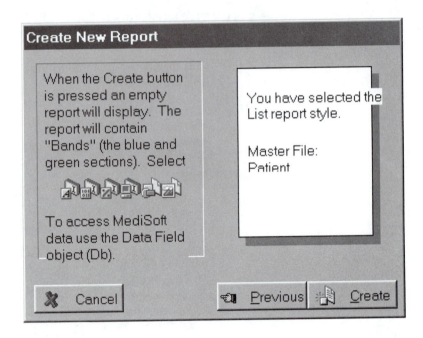

- Click create, and the following screen appears, called the **report designer grid**. On the grid the user indicates what fields data should be taken from, as well as static text fields, where the fields (from which files) should be placed on the report, and the format of the text. All changes to design are made on this grid.

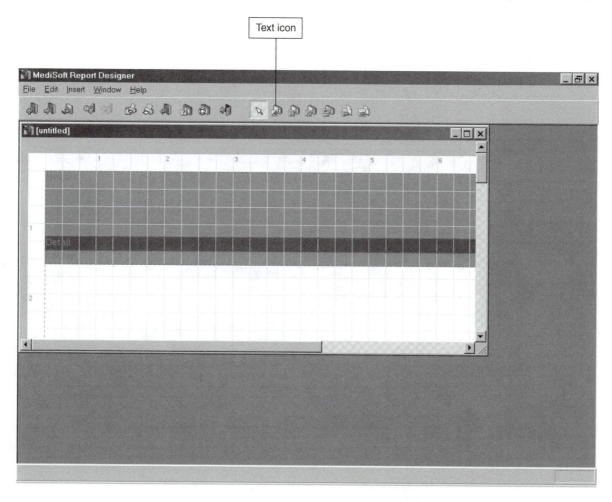

Text icon

- Click on the text icon on the toolbar.
- Click in the **header** area of the report designer grid, and a text box will appear on the grid. Headers are text.
- Double-click on the text box and the following dialog box will appear. Enter the title (patient report) and click OK.

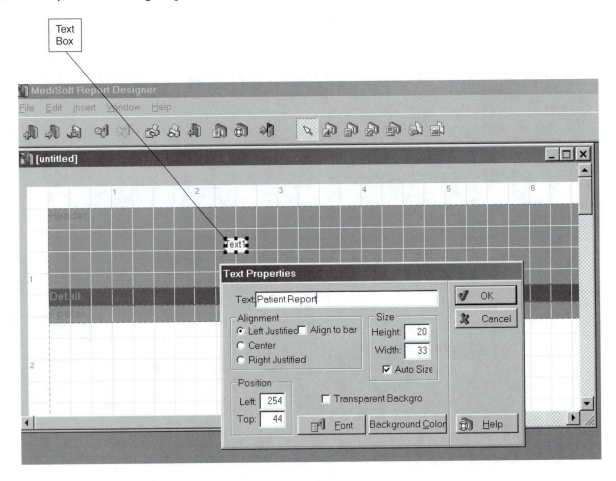

To add detail lines (the lines of actual data) which will appear many times in the report:

- Click on the data field icon, and on the detail area of the grid. A data field box appears on the report on the detail line.

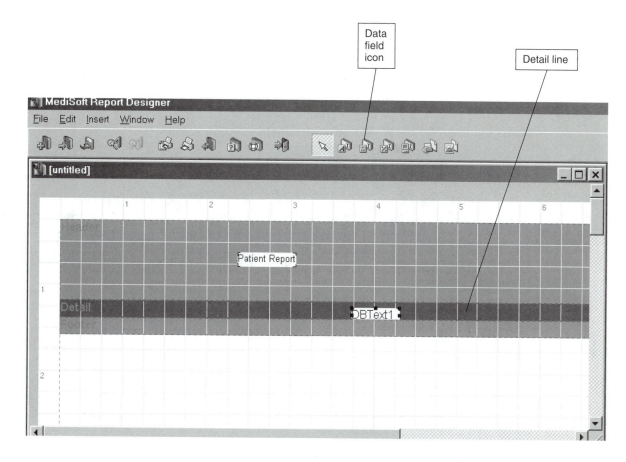

- Double-click on the detail data field box, and the following dialog box will be displayed.

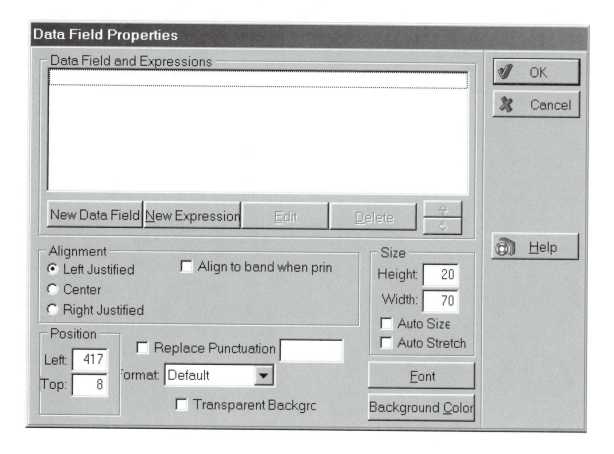

- When a data field is chosen, you must click new data field in the above dialog box. The following list of files and fields is displayed:

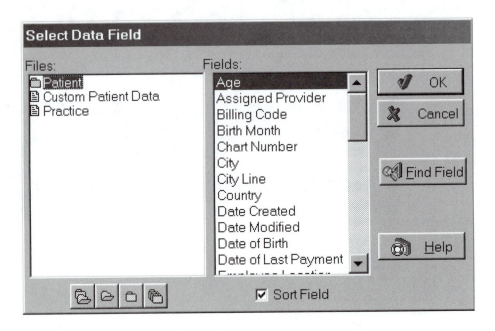

- You can see that it displays file names and field names from your database. First choose the file (patients) and then choose a field to appear in the report; the *contents* of the field will be displayed in the finished report.

- Scroll down until you see full name (LFM). Double-click on it, and the data field properties dialog box appears.

- Fill in the alignment option you want (left).

- Click OK.

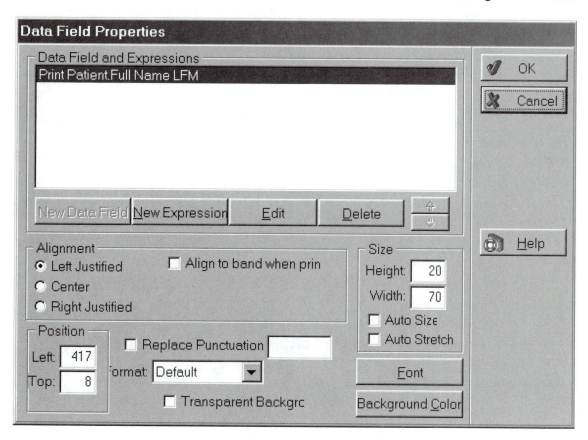

- Repeat this process to select the next field (chart number). Remember to double-click on the data field box and click new field in the next dialog box. Choose chart number from the list and click OK.

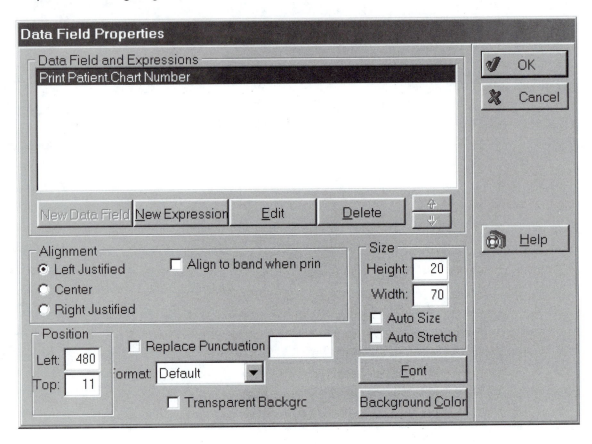

On your own, add assigned provider as a data field in the detail area. Add column headers in the header area for name (click on text, click on header where you want the header, double-click the text box, fill in the text, click OK), chart number (text), and provider (text). In addition, add a third data field (click on the data field icon, click in the detail area where you want the field, double-click the box on the grid, click new data field, and select the field provider from the list of fields, then click OK).

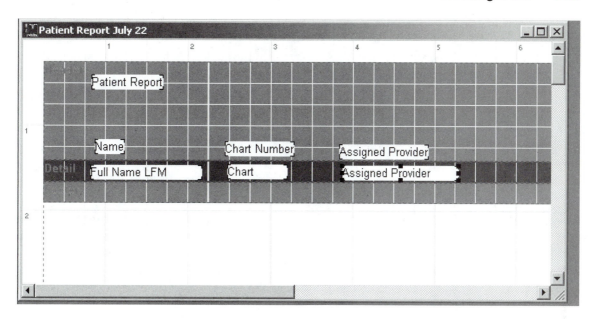

Add a **footer** by clicking on the text icon, clicking in the footer area. When the text box appears, double-click on it. In the text properties dialog box, enter Created by Your Name. To change the font to 9 point, click on the font command button and select 9 as the size. Click OK, and click OK again.

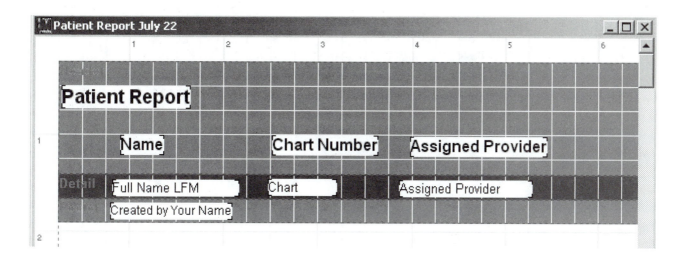

You can change the size and style of the text by right-clicking on the text, and choosing properties. For each column header, choose bold as the style and 12 as the font size. Click OK and click OK again. Each title needs to be done separately. The report title (Patient Report) should be bold and 14 point.

Click on the preview report icon. Save the report as patient report and click OK. Click on preview again. The report you designed should resemble this:

Patient Report

Name	Chart Number	Assigned Provider
Again, Dwight	AGADW	REL
Austin, Andrew	AUBAN0	JM
Bordon, John	BORJO0	JM
Brimley, Jay	BRIJA00	MM
Brimley, Susan	BRISU00	MM
Brown, Tonya	BROTO0	MM
Catera, Samuel	CATSC0	MM
Clinger, Wallace	CLIWI00	
Doe, Jane S	DOEJA0	JM
Doogan, James	DOOJA0	
Gooding, Charles	GOOCH0	
Green, Jenna	GREJE0	MM
Hartman, Tonya	HARTO0	
Jasper, Stephanie L	JASST0	
Jones, Suzy Q	JONSU0	REL
Karvel, Jessica C	KARJE0	
Lewis, Monique	LEWMO	
Patel, Kathy I	PATKA0	JM
Wagnew, Jeremy	WAGJE	JM
Youngblood,	YOUMI0	WH
Zimmerman,	ZIMAN00	

You may not see the footer on the screen; however, you will see it on the printed page. Print the report.

If you do not like the appearance of the report, for example, if headers look out-of-line, you can move any object around by closing the preview window and clicking on the object (e.g., text box) and dragging it around on the **custom report grid**. Its formatting can be changed by pointing to the object, right-clicking, and choosing properties.

CREATING A LABELS REPORT

To create a labels report, pull down the file menu and choose new. Choose label.

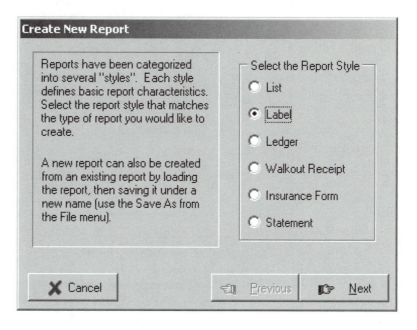

Click next.

In the next dialog box, select address as the file from which to take data. Click Next.

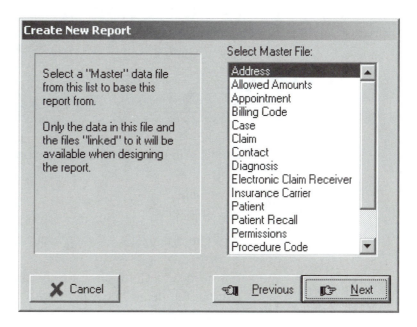

In the dialog box that opens, choose three columns across.

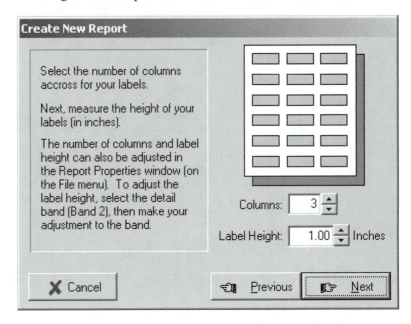

Click next. And on the next screen click create.

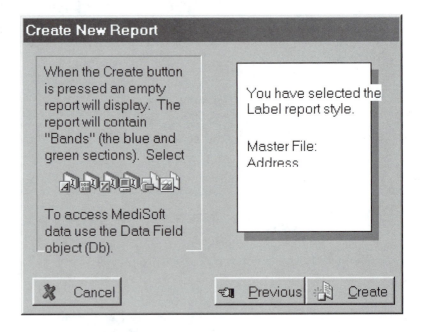

On the grid that is displayed, you are going to add data fields for:

Name
Street1
City State ZIP

For each data field, click on the data field icon on the toolbar, then click in the detail line where you want it to appear. Double-click the data field box, click new field, choose the field from the list, and click OK. If you want to, try to add a comma between city and state—it is a text field.

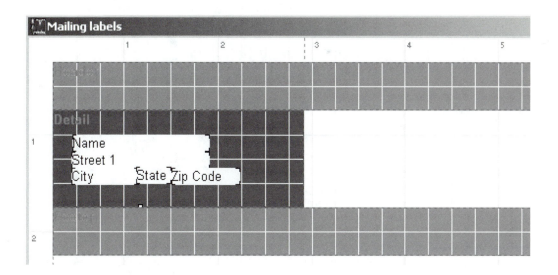

Preview the report. Save it as mailing labels. If you do not like the way it looks, close the preview screen and move the field names around on the grid until you like the appearance.

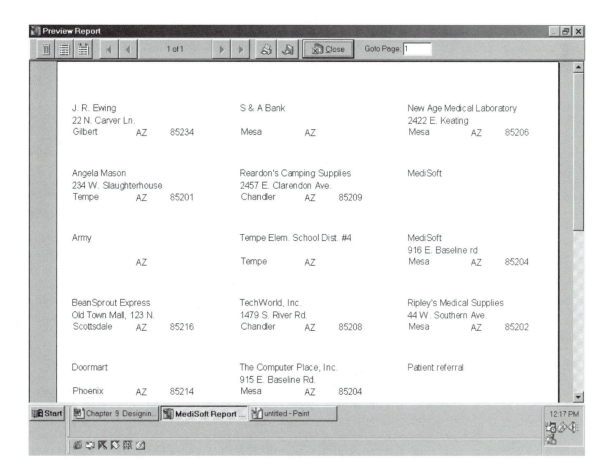

CREATING A CUSTOM LEDGER REPORT

To create a report in **ledger** style, pull down the reports menu and select design custom reports and bills. Click the new icon on the report designer toolbar.

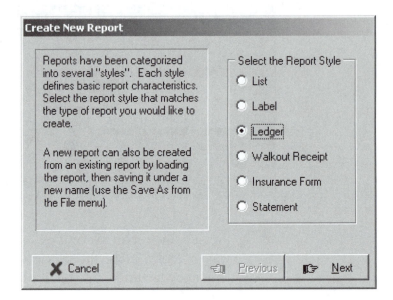

Select ledger and click next. In the dialog box that opens, select patient as the master file.

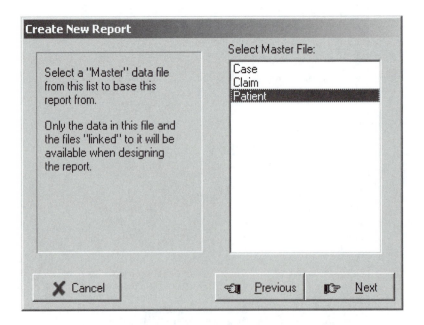

Click next.

In the next dialog box that opens, select case as the detail file. Click next.

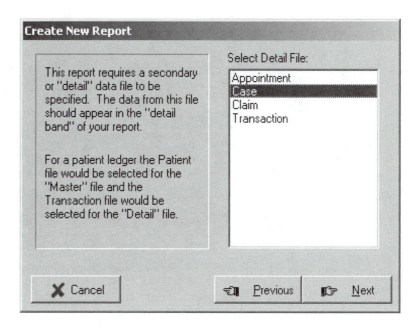

Click next.

The following window should be displayed:

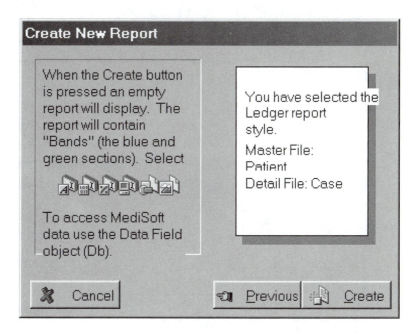

Click create and the following screen should be displayed:

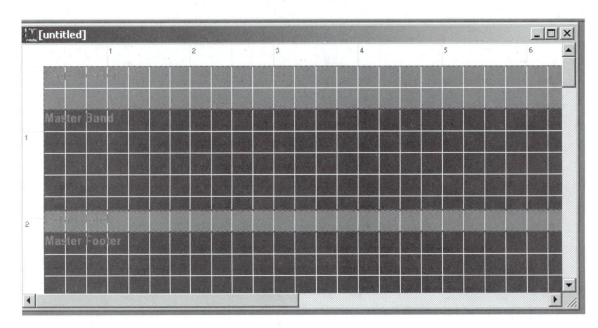

Click on the data field icon on the toolbar and click in the master band section of the screen. A text box will appear. Double-click on the box, and the following window opens:

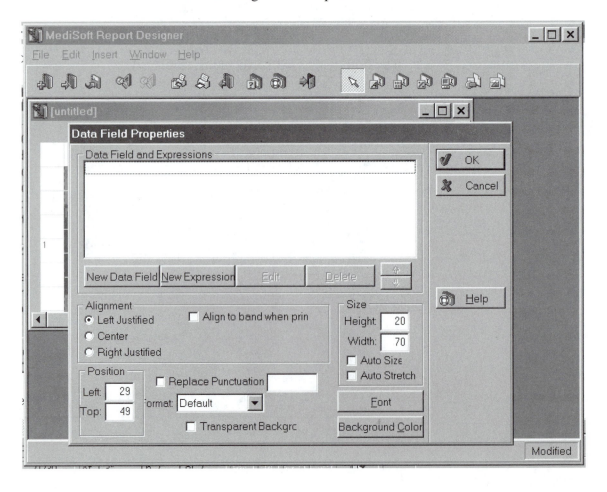

Click the new data field command button. Select patient as the file.

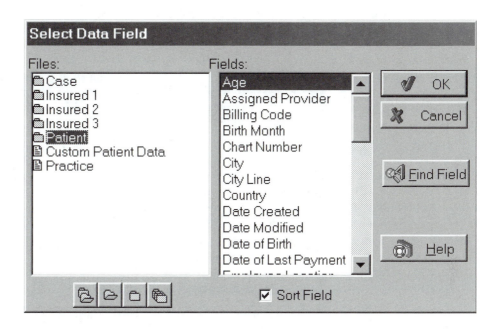

Choose patient full name (LFM) as the data field. Click OK. In the data field properties window, click OK.

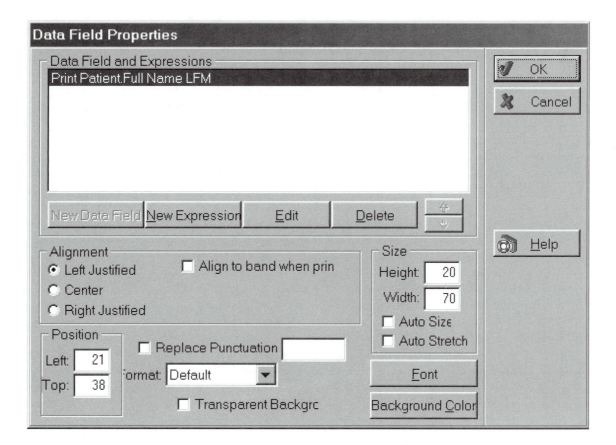

To add detail lines, click on the data field icon, then click in the detail band. Double-click on the text box that opens. Choose case as the file and diagnosis 1 as the data field.

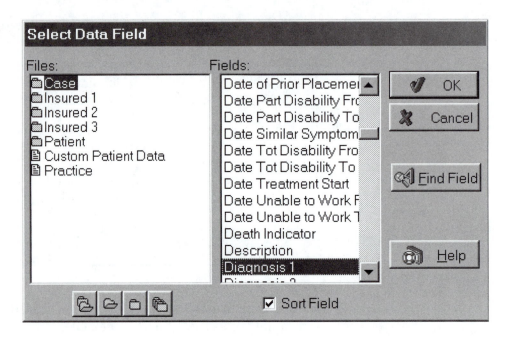

Click OK. In the dialog box that opens, click new data item and click OK. Click OK again.

On your own, add print patient statements as a data field in the detail band.

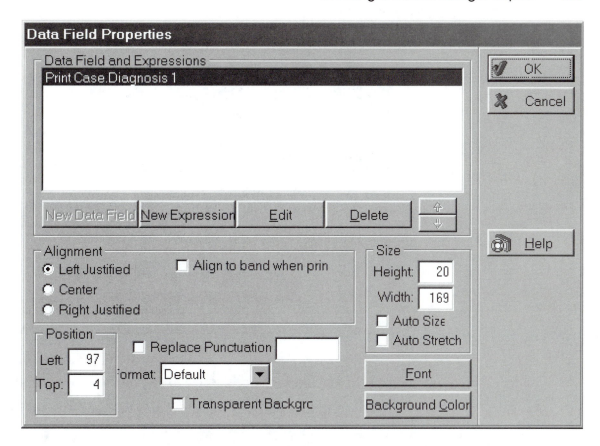

Add a page footer with the following text, then click OK.

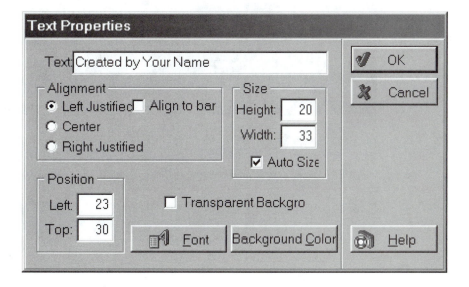

Add a report title:

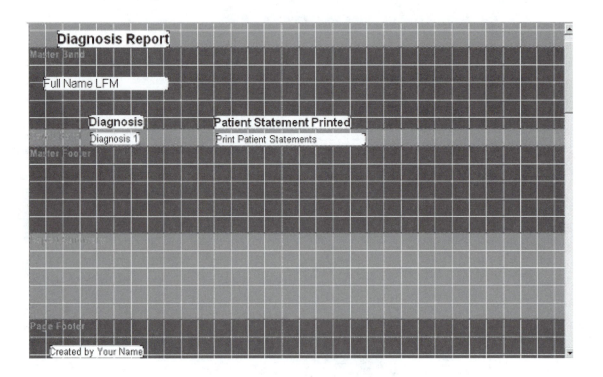

Click on font, then change the size to 16 point and the style to bold.

Add the following column headers in the header area (both text fields): diagnosis (bold, 12 point) and patient statement printed (bold, 12 point). In the detail band, add a data field (print patient statement). Preview the report. Save the report as diagnosis report, and click

OK. Click the preview icon again. The report should resemble the following:

Diagnosis Report

Açain, Dwight

Diagnosis	Patient Statement Printed
959.4	True
847.2	True
C34.0	True
724.2	True
724.2	True

Acsin, Andrew

Diagnosis	Patient Statement Printed
V700	True

Print the report.

You do not need to create walkout receipts or insurance forms or statements because MediSoft has a custom designed walkout receipt and many statements. However, you can create your own statements and insurance forms using the report designer.

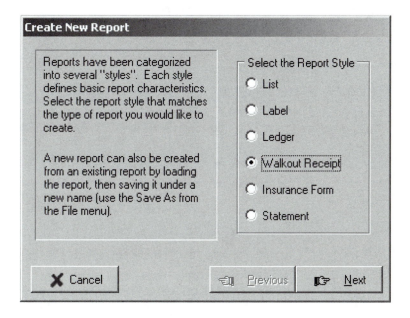

Chapter Summary

- MediSoft allows the user to design custom reports and statements.
- The user may choose the style from a dialog box: list, label, ledger, walkout receipt, insurance form, or statement.
- The user utilizes the custom design grid to arrange and format text and fields from one or more tables.

Key Words

Custom report grid
Data fields
Detail
Detail line
Footer

Header
Ledger
Report designer
Report designer grid

REVIEW EXERCISES

Define the following terms:

Data field

Detail line

Footer

Header

Identify the buttons on the report designer toolbar by filling in the empty boxes:

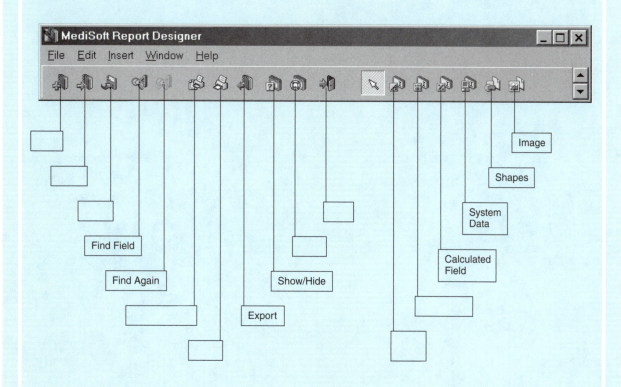

10 Setting up a New Practice

Chapter Outline

Learning Objectives

After completing this chapter, the student will be able to establish a new practice database using MediSoft, including:

- Making the practice HIPAA compliant
- Entering practice information
- Entering provider information
- Entering address information
- Entering patient information
- Entering insurance carriers

- Entering diagnosis codes
- Entering billing codes
- Entering procedure, payment, and adjustment codes
- Entering and editing patients and cases
- Entering transactions and creating claims
- Generating reports
- Viewing the deposit list

HIPAA COMPLIANCE

MediSoft (after Version 6) allows you to choose options that make your program comply with the Health Insurance Portability and Accountability Act (1996), which set privacy standards for patient information. Pull down the file menu and choose program options. Click on the HIPAA tab and click on auto log off and warn on unapproved codes. Once a user is logged off, she or he will need a password to log back into the program; this helps guard against unauthorized use of the program and protects privacy. Click the save command button.

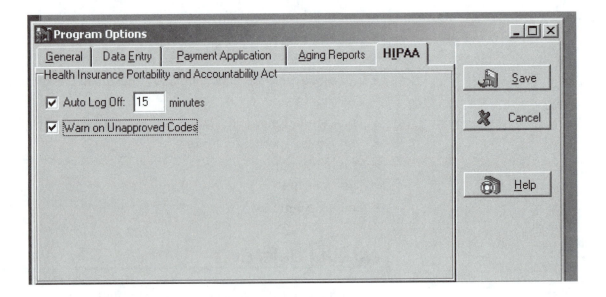

ENTERING PRACTICE INFORMATION

If you are starting a practice or computerizing an existing practice using MediSoft, there are several tasks you need to complete. To set up a new database file, do the following:

• Pull down the File menu and choose new practice.

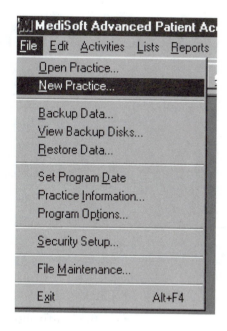

The following dialog box will be displayed:

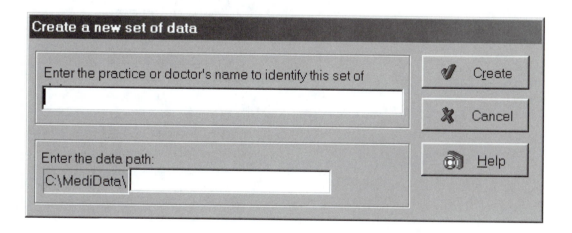

• Enter the practice name (Dr. Phyllis Malloy). You need to create a folder for the database. Your data path will be C:\MediData\Malloy.

- Enter Malloy in the enter the data path text box.

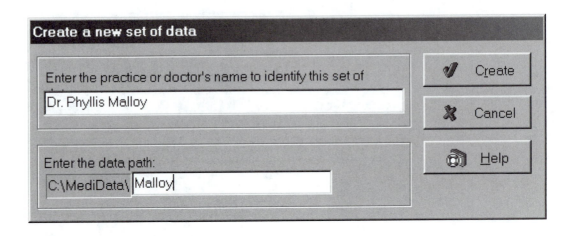

- Click create.
- In the confirm dialog box that opens, click yes.

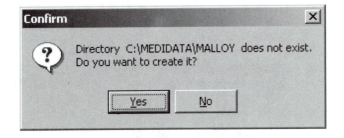

The following dialog box will be displayed:

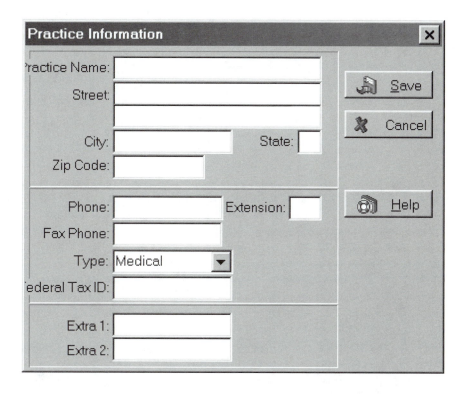

• Fill in Dr. Malloy's practice information as presented below and save the record.

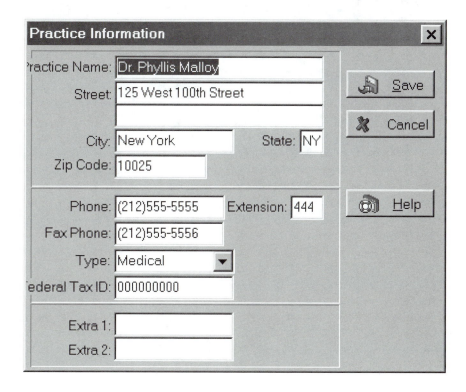

ENTERING PROVIDER INFORMATION

Next, you need to enter provider information for Dr. Malloy. To enter provider information, do the following:

- Pull down the lists menu and click provider.
- Click new.
- Add the following information:

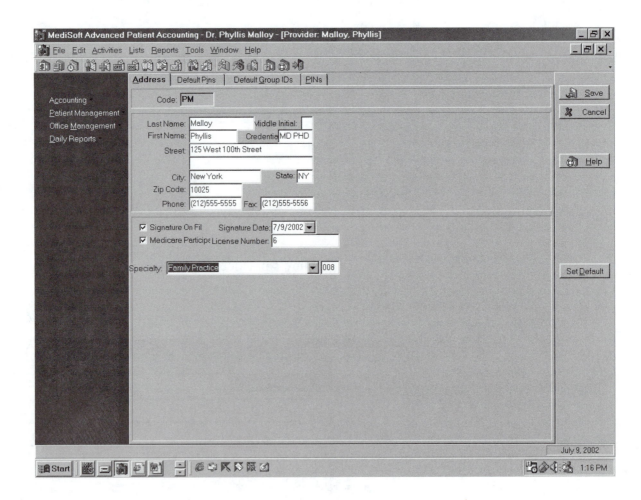

- Click the default PINs tab (under the toolbar) and enter the following:

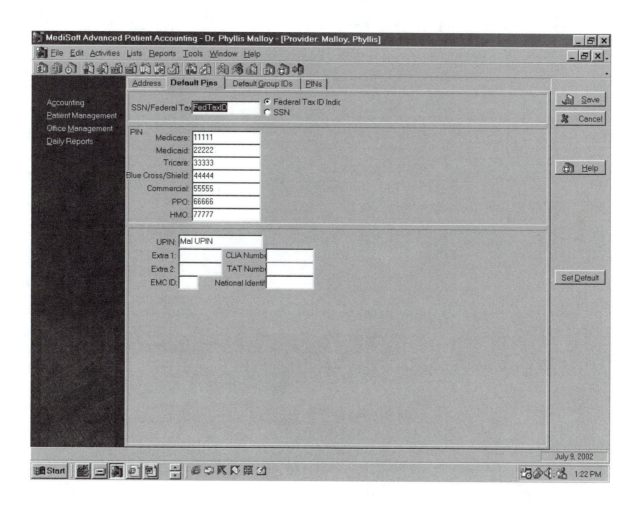

ENTERING ADDRESS INFORMATION

It is necessary to enter information in the address list. Either click on the address icon on the toolbar or pull down the lists menu and choose addresses. Click the new command button. In the dialog box that opens, tab over the code to the name field, and enter the following information and choose miscellaneous from the drop-down list:

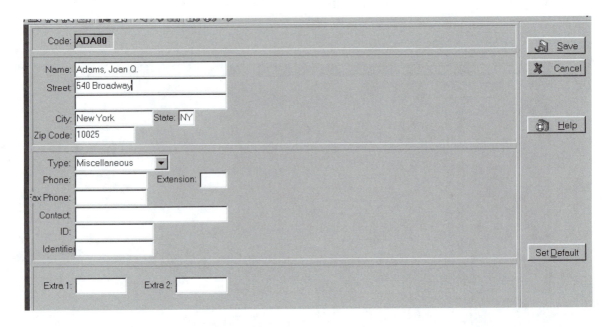

- Save the record. The information will appear on the address list.
- Perform the same steps to enter the rest of the patients' addresses.

Add the following to the address list. Each type is miscellaneous.

Santiago, Rose
135 East 102nd Street
New York, NY 10025

Shah, James
345 Amsterdam Avenue
New York, NY 10025

Wang, Amy
444 Central Park West
New York, NY 10025

Wang, Karen
444 Central Park West
New York, NY 10025

Williams, Franklin D.
125 Columbus Avenue
New York, NY 10025

Add a record for yourself. Be sure to save after adding each record.

Now you need to enter employer information on the address list. Enter the following:

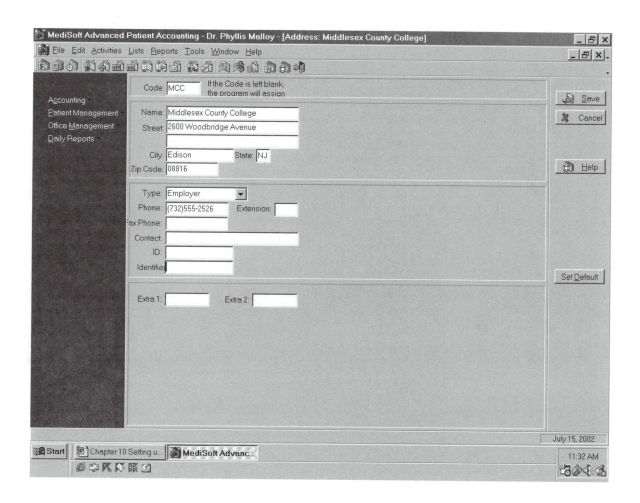

Enter a second employer:

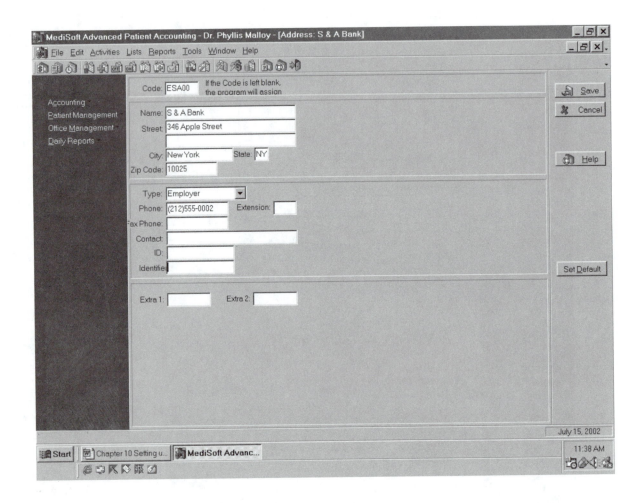

Add a third employer:

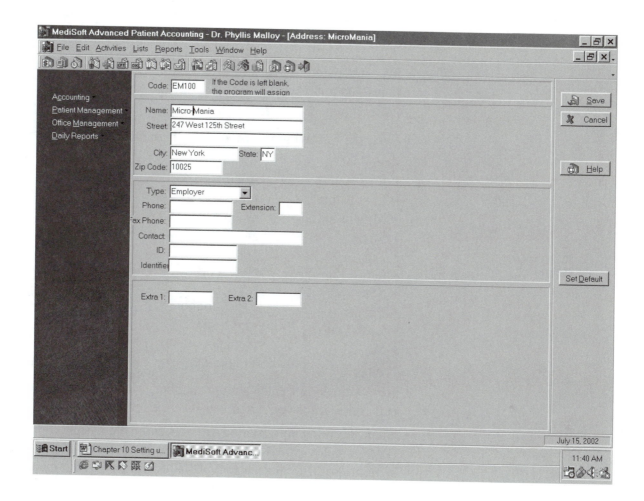

After saving this information, your address list should resemble this:

Code	Name	Phone	Type	Extension
ADA00	Adams, Joan Q.		Miscellaneous	
EM100	Micro-Mania		Employer	
ESA00	S & A Bank	(212)555-0002	Employer	
MCC	Middlesex County Colleg	(732)555-2526	Employer	
SAN00	Santiago, Rosa		Miscellaneous	
SHA00	Shah, James		Miscellaneous	
WAN00	Wang, Amy		Miscellaneous	
WAN01	Wang, Karen		Miscellaneous	
WIL00	Williams, Franklin D.		Miscellaneous	

ENTERING PATIENT INFORMATION

You need to enter a list of patients that use Dr. Malloy's practice. Do the following:

- To enter patient data, pull down the lists menu and choose patients/guarantors and cases.
- Click new.
- Enter the following information in the name, address page of the dialog box:
  - Last Name   Adams
  - First Name   Joan
  - Middle Initial   Q
  - Street   540 Broadway
  - Zip   10025
  - City   New York
  - State   NY
  - Phone   2125559999
  - Birth Date   5/25/1946
  - Sex   Female
  - SSN   111111111
- However, do not enter a chart number. MediSoft will automatically enter it for you when you save the record.
- Click the other information tab and enter the assigned provider (PM), employer (MCC), employment status (part time). Check signature on file and enter 5/10/79 as the date. This means she will not have to sign each insurance form.
- Save the record.
- You will be brought back to the patient list.

- Click new to add a new patient.
- Enter the following information in the name, address page of the dialog box:
  - Last Name   Williams
  - First Name   Franklin
  - Middle Initial   D
  - Street   125 Columbus Avenue
  - Zip   10025
  - City   New York
  - State   NY
  - Phone   2125557777
  - Birth Date   2/7/1953
  - Sex   Male
  - SSN   333333333

- Click the other information tab and enter the assigned provider (PM). His employer is Micro-Mania, and he is employed full time. Check signature on file and enter 2/10/95 as the date.
- Save the record, and MediSoft assigns a chart number.

- Click new to add a third patient:
- Enter the following information in the name, address page of the dialog box.
  - Last Name   Shah
  - First Name   James
  - Middle Initial
  - Street   343 Amsterdam Avenue
  - Zip   10025
  - City   New York
  - State   NY
  - Phone   2125552222
  - Birth Date   7/14/1960
  - Sex   Male
  - SSN   222222222
- Click the other information tab and enter the assigned provider (PM). His employer is the S&A Bank; he is employed full time. Check signature on file and enter 2/10/85 as the date.
- Save the record and MediSoft assigns a chart number.

- Click new to add another patient.
- Enter the following information on the name, address page of the dialog box.
  - Last Name   Cohen
  - First Name   Miriam
  - Middle Initial   B
  - Street   785 West End Avenue
  - Zip   10025
  - City   New York
  - State   NY
  - Phone   2125556710
  - Birth Date   5/7/1937
  - Sex   Female
  - SSN   555555555
- Click the other information tab and enter the assigned provider (PM). Check signature on file and enter 5/10/55 as the date.
- Save the record and MediSoft assigns a chart number.

- Click new.

- Enter the following information in the name, address page of the dialog box.
  - Last Name   Santiago
  - First Name   Rosa
  - Middle Initial
  - Street   135 East 102 Street
  - Zip   10015
  - City   New York
  - State   NY
  - Phone   2125558888
  - Birth Date   9/6/1973
  - Sex   Female
  - SSN   444444444
- Click the other information tab and enter the assigned provider (PM).
- Save the record.

- Then, add patients with the following information:
- Click new (before entering each patient's record).
- Enter the following information in the name, address page of the dialog box.
  - Last Name   Wang
  - First Name   Amy
  - Middle Initial
  - Street   444 Central Park West
  - Zip   10025
  - City   New York
  - State   NY
  - Phone   2125550000
  - Birth Date   7/25/2001
  - Sex   Female
  - SSN   666666666
- Click the other information tab and enter the assigned provider (PM).
- Save the record.

- Click new.
- Enter the following information in the name, address page of the dialog box.
  - Last Name   Wang
  - First Name   Karen
  - Middle Initial
  - Street   444 Central Park West
  - Zip   10025
  - City   New York
  - State   NY

- Phone   2125550000
- Birth Date   5/3/1970
- Sex   Female
- SSN   777777777

- Click the other information tab and enter the assigned provider (PM). Check signature on file and enter 3/30/95 as the date.

- Save the record.

- Click new and add a record for yourself as a patient. Include your real name. Your provider is Dr. Malloy. You can make up the rest of the information. Save the record.

The patient list should resemble the following with the additional record for yourself:

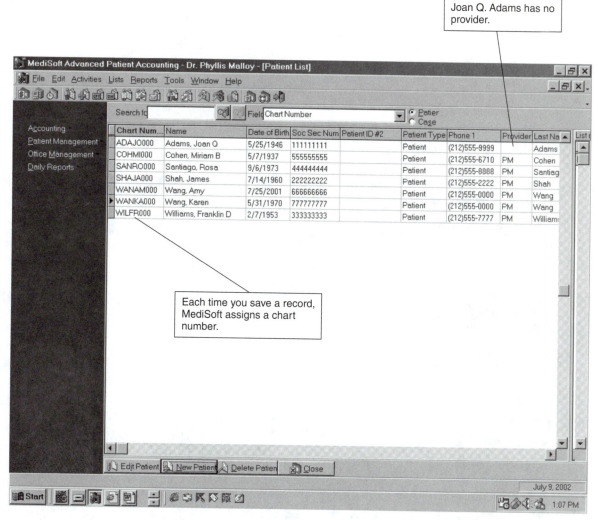

Joan Q. Adams has no provider.

Each time you save a record, MediSoft assigns a chart number.

Note that Joan Q. Adams has no provider assigned. Edit her record by double-clicking on her name and clicking the other information tab. Enter PM as her provider.

ENTERING INSURANCE CARRIERS

You also need to create a list of insurance carriers.

• Pull down the lists menu and choose insurance carriers.

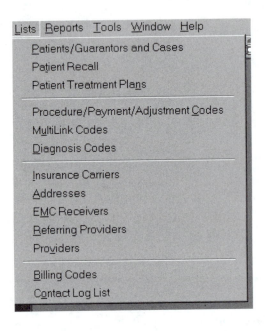

In the dialog box that opens,

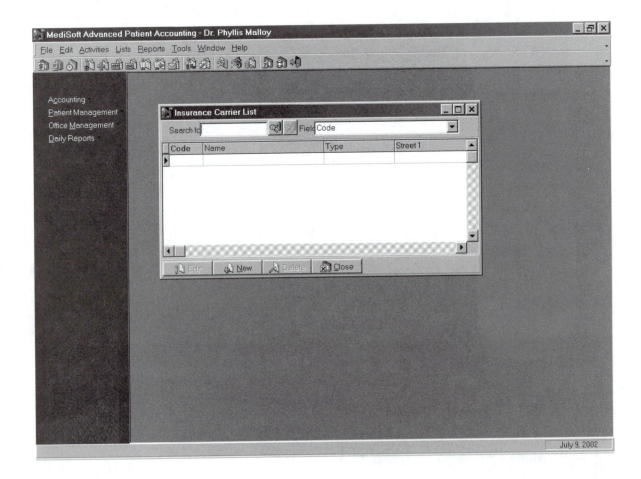

- Click new.
- Add the following information:
  - Name   Aetna
  - Address   PO Box 960
  - City   Bluebell
  - State   PA
  - Zip   19422
  - Phone   8005551122
  - Extension   4
  - Fax   8005551123
  - Contact   Jane Smith
- Click the options tab. Click the down-arrow next to type and select HMO.
- Save the record and MediSoft assigns a code.

- Click new.
- Add a second carrier with the following information:
  - Name   Blue Cross/Blue Shield
  - Address   88 Broad Street
  - City   Philadelphia
  - State   PA
  - Zip   17109
  - Phone   2155559089
  - Extension   49
  - Fax   2155559088
  - Contact
- Click the options tab. Click the down-arrow next to type and select Blue Cross/Blue Shield.
- Save the record and MediSoft assigns a code.

- Click new.
- Add a third carrier with the following information:
  - Name   Medicaid
  - Address   123 Broadway
  - City   New York
  - State   NY
  - Zip   10025
  - Phone   2125555675
  - Extension   49
  - Fax   2125559088
  - Contact
- Click the options tab. Click the down-arrow next to type and select Medicaid.
- Save the record and MediSoft assigns a code.

- Click new.
- Add a carrier with the following information:
  - Name   Medicare
  - Address   89 Main Street
  - City   Newark
  - State   NJ
  - Zip   06000
  - Phone   2735554321
  - Extension   6789
  - Fax   2735554322
  - Contact
- Click the options tab. Click the down-arrow next to type and select Medicare.
- Save the record and MediSoft assigns a code.
- Remember to click new before each carrier.
- Add carriers with the following information:
  - Name   Cigna
  - Address   123 West 73rd Street
  - City   New York
  - State   NY
  - Zip   10025
  - Phone   2125555675
  - Extension
  - Fax   2125555678
  - Contact
- Click the options tab. Click the down-arrow next to type and select HMO.
- Save the record and MediSoft assigns a code.

- Click new.
  - Name   Worker's Compensation
  - Address   1 Delaware Street
  - City   Washington
  - State   DC
  - Zip   30000
  - Phone   8005551074
  - Extension
  - Fax   8005551075
  - Contact
- Click the options tab. Click the down-arrow next to type and select Worker's Comp.
- Save the record and MediSoft assigns a code.

Your insurance carrier list should resemble the following:

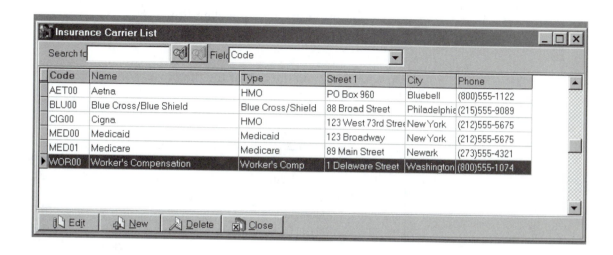

ENTERING DIAGNOSIS CODES

You now need to add a list of the diagnoses common to Dr. Malloy's practice. To add a diagnosis list, do the following:

- Pull down lists and choose diagnosis codes. Diagnosis codes are added one at a time.
- Click new and fill in the following information:
  - Code 1   034.0
  - Description   Strep Throat
- Save the record.

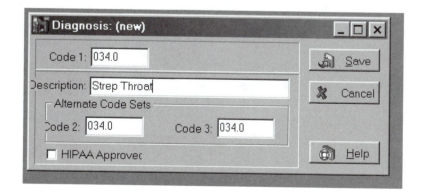

• Click new and fill in the following information to add a second diagnosis code:

    • Code 1   052.9
    • Description   Chicken Pox

• Save the record.

On your own, add the rest of the diagnosis codes:

Code 1	Description	Code 2	Code 3
034.0	Strep Throat	034.0	034.0
052.9	Chicken Pox	052.9	052.9
075.0	Mononucleosis	075.0	075.0
250.01	IDDM Diabetes Mellitis	250.01	250.01
346.9	Headache-Migraine	346.9	346.9
401.9	Hypertension	401.9	401.9
422.9	Heart Disease	422.9	422.9
465.9	Upper Respiratory Infection	465.9	465.9
724.2	Low Back Pain	724.2	724.2

ENTERING BILLING CODES

To enter **billing codes** do the following:

• Pull down the lists menu and select billing codes.
• Click the new command button before entering each code and save after each entry.
• Add the following codes:

Co...	Description
A	Default Billing Code
C	Cash Patient
GY	GYN Patient
H	HMO Patient
M	Medicare Patient
NS	Non-smoker
OB	OB Patient
P	PPO Patient
S	Smoker

ENTERING PROCEDURE, PAYMENT, AND ADJUSTMENT CODES

A list of procedure, payment, and adjustment codes also needs to be entered. Because there are several types of codes on this list, you must be very careful to correctly identify the type of each code as a charge, a payment, an adjustment, or a procedure. To add procedure and payment codes, do the following:

- Click on the CPT icon or pull down the lists menu and select procedure, payment, and adjustment list. Click new. A three-tabbed dialog box is displayed. You will need to fill in information on each page of the dialog box for each code.

- Enter 36215 as Code 1.

- Enter lab drawing fee as the description.

- Enter inside lab charge as the code type (select it using the drop-down arrow in the code type drop-down list box).

- Enter 5 as type of service.

- Enter 0 as time to do procedure.

- Enter A as service classification.

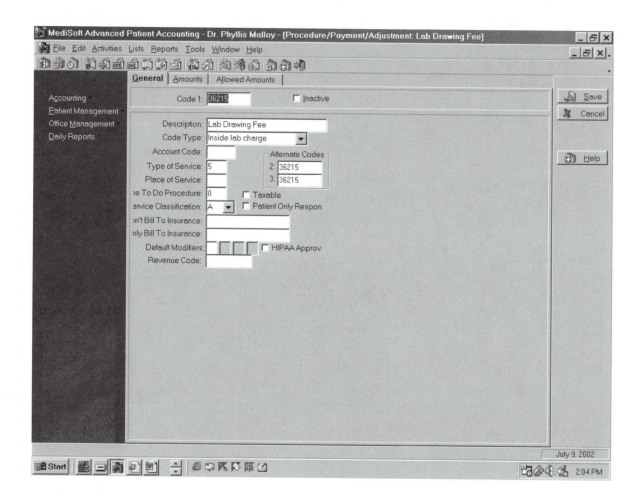

• Click on the amounts tab and enter 8 as charge amount A.

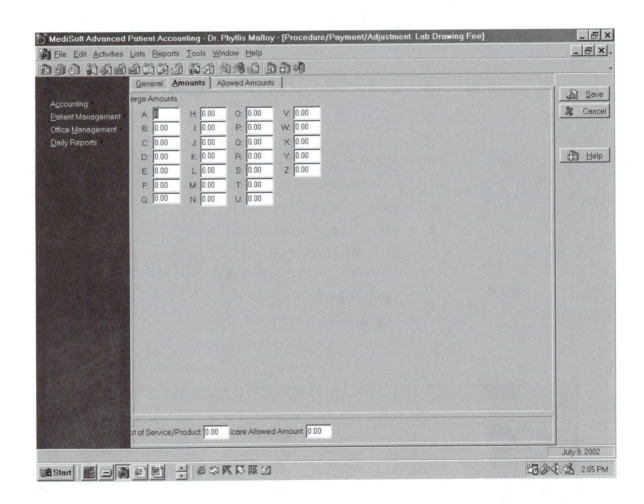

• Click on allowed amounts tab and enter the following information:

Insurance Name	Code	Modifiers	Amount
Aetna	AET00		7.50
Blue Cross/Blue Shield	BLU00		7.50
Cigna	CIG00		7.00
Medicaid	MED00		4.00
Medicare	MED01		6.45
Worker's Compensation	WOR00		6.00

• Save the record.

- Add the rest of the information. Be very careful to enter the correct type.

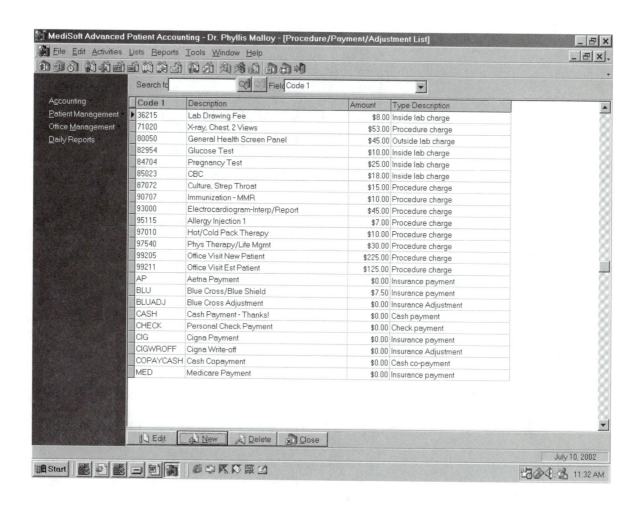

To simplify this exercise, only enter amount and allowed amount for the codes we will use. As you know, the amount refers to the price charged for the service by the practice. The allowed amount is the basis on which the insurance company calculates the amount of money it will pay the practice for the service. For example, it may pay 80 percent of the allowed amount. MediSoft uses the allowed amount to calculate insurance responsibility, patient responsibility, and adjustments. The 20 percent—the difference between the allowed amount and the insurance payment—is the patient's responsibility. The difference between the allowed amount and the charge is written off by the practice. Adjustments and write-offs are also entered on this list. An adjustment is a positive or negative change in a patient's charge. If an account is sent to a collection agency, the adjustment would add to the patient's amount owed. An adjustment is entered in the same way as a payment, and needs to be applied to the patient's account. For general health screen, enter 45.00 as the charge amount and the following as allowed amounts. Pull down the lists menu, choose procedures/payment/adjustment, double-click on general health screen, and enter the following:

General	Amounts	Allowed Amounts			
Insurance Name			Code	Modifiers	Amount
Aetna			AET00		35.00
Blue Cross/Blue Shield			BLU00		35.00
Cigna			CIG00		35.00
Medicaid			MED00		20.00
Medicare			MED01		30.00
Worker's Compensation			WOR00		20.00

You will see later that Karen Wang was charged 45.00 for a General Health Screen Panel, insurance paid 35.00, and the practice wrote off (adjusted her account down) 10.00.

- For the lab drawing fee, enter 8.00 as the charge, and the following as allowed amounts:

General	Amounts	Allowed Amounts			
Insurance Name			Code	Modifiers	Amount
Aetna			AET00		7.50
Blue Cross Blue Shield 231			BLU00		7.50
Cigna			CIG00		7.00
Medicaid			MED00		4.00
Medicare			MED01		6.45
Worker's Compensation			WOR00		6.00

Fill in 15.00 as amount charged for a strep culture, and the following allowed amounts:

General	Amounts	Allowed Amounts			
Insurance Name			Code	Modifiers	Amount
Aetna			AET00		15.00
Blue Cross/Blue Shield			BLU00		15.00
Cigna			CIG00		10.00
Medicaid			MED00		5.00
Medicare			MED01		9.00
Worker's Compensation			WOR00		12.00

ENTERING CASES

Enter a new case for Joan Q. Adams by doing the following:

- Pull down the lists menu and select patients/guarantors and cases.
- Click on Joan Q. Adams and click the case option button.
- Click the new command button.
- Click on the personal tab.

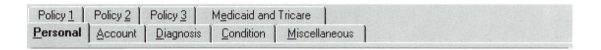

Only the chart number and guarantor are filled in by MediSoft.

- Fill in the information below:

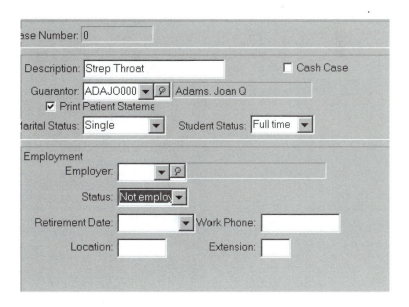

- Click on the account tab and click on the arrow in the provider drop-down list box and select Dr. Malloy.

- Click on the diagnosis tab and select strep throat from the default diagnosis 1 drop-down list.

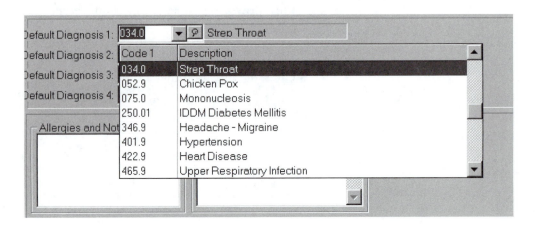

- Click on the condition tab and fill in the following information by selecting from drop-down lists or typing it.

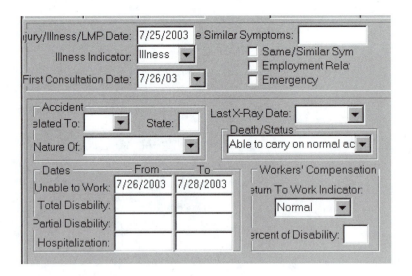

• Click on the policy 1 tab and enter the following:

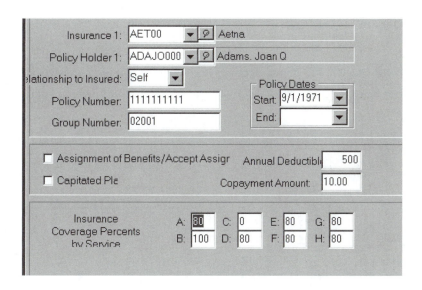

• Click on the save command button on the upper right corner of the screen.

TRANSACTION ENTRY AND CLAIM MANAGEMENT

To enter transactions in the old style, pull down the file menu and select program options, click on the data entry tab, and click on use old style transactions.

• Pull down the activities menu and select enter transactions.

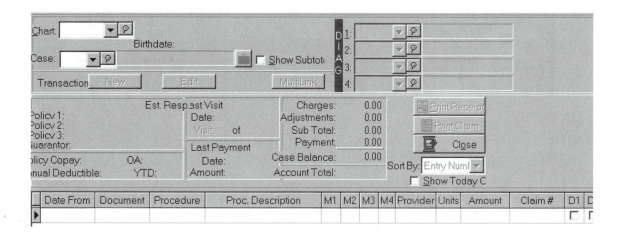

- Click on the down arrow of the chart number drop-down list box, and select Joan Q. Adams.

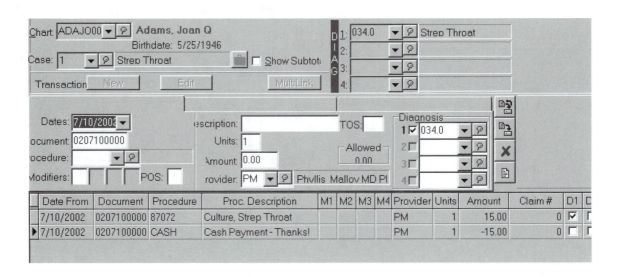

- Click the new command button.
- Click on the charges tab.
- In the dialog box that opens, select a procedure code for culture, strep throat from the drop-down list box.
- Enter the following:

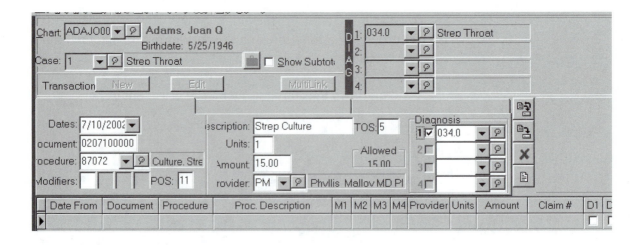

- Save the transaction entry.
- Click new.
- Click the payment tab.
- Enter the Pay Code: CASH

- Click the drop-down arrow in the who paid? dialog box and select Joan Q. Adams.

- Enter check as payment description.

- Enter 15.00 as amount paid.

- Select Dr. Malloy as provider.

- Press enter.

- Click on apply payment to charges. (It will automatically appear on the deposit list after the record is saved.)

- In the dialog box that appears enter –15.00.

- Close the window. Click on save.

After all the information has been entered, Joan Q. Adams's transaction looks like this:

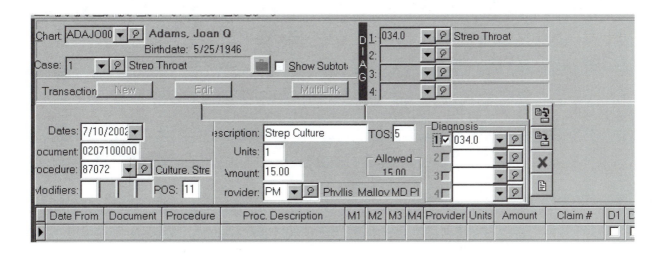

If a message appears saying that the data is not entered, create data now, click OK.

Enter a new case for Miriam Cohen. On July 10, 2003, Miriam attempted to remove an air conditioner and suffered severe back spasms. She was given an emergency appointment with Dr. Malloy.

Click on the office hours icon on the toolbar. Double-click the space next to 8:15a, and enter the following:

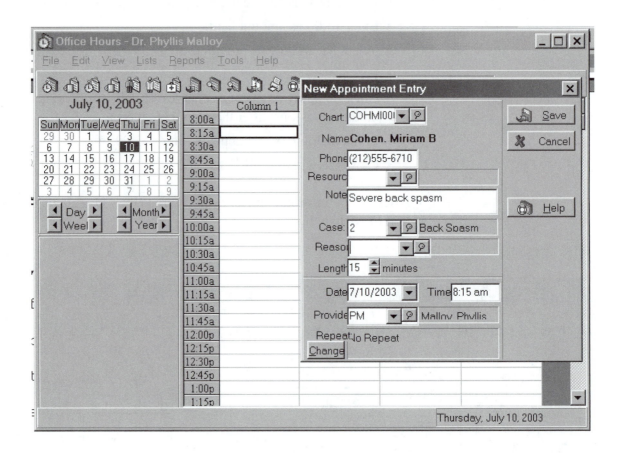

Enter the case (back spasm) by clicking on the down-arrow and selecting from the drop-down list. Close Office Hours. Pull down the lists menu and select patients/guarantors and cases. Click on Miriam Cohen and click the cases option button. Click new and fill in the following information on the personal tab:

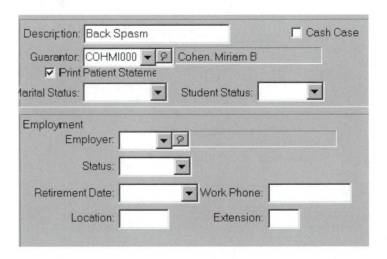

Click on the policy 1 tab and enter the following:

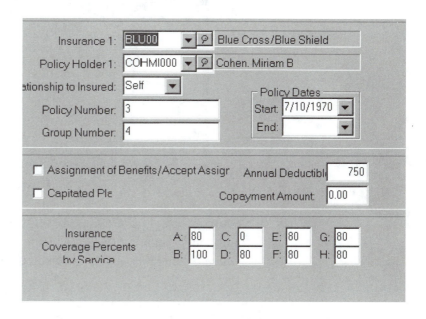

Click the account tab and fill in PM as the provider. Click the diagnosis 1 tab and fill in low back pain. Click the condition tab and fill in Back Spasms as the Illness Indicator and illness as the Illness. The first consultation date is 7/7/2003 and the dates unable to work are 7/7/2003 to 7/17/2003.

To enter a transaction for Miriam Cohen (a charge of 10.00), pull down the activities menu and choose enter transactions. Fill in COHMI000; click new; make sure the charge tab is selected. Enter low back pain as the description. The amount is filled in automatically. Save the transaction. The second transaction is a cash payment by Ms. Cohen of 2.50. This is a new transaction (remember to click new). Make sure the payment tab is selected. Enter a cash payment by Miriam Cohen of 2.50 and apply the payment to the charge. Print a receipt for her by clicking the print receipt button. Next we will create a claim to be sent to her insurance company. Her insurance must be billed for the remainder of the payment. You can create a claim for her either from the transaction screen by clicking on print claim or from claim management. MediSoft will not allow the creation of duplicate claims. Click print claim, choose HCFA summary, click start. You will see the claim on the screen and receive the message that one claim has been created. If you need to edit the claim, highlight the claim in the claim management window and click edit. You can check the status of your claims at the claim management window. The claim is ready to send.

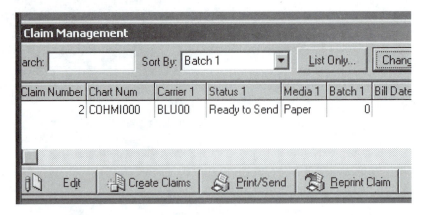

You can change the status to sent by clicking on the change status button and changing the status from ready to send to sent. In addition, you can change the status to rejected, challenged, and so on.

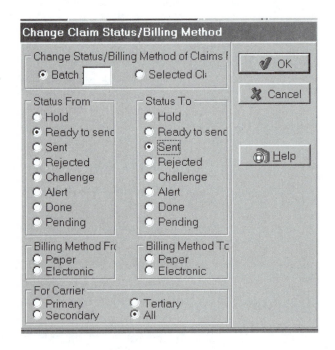

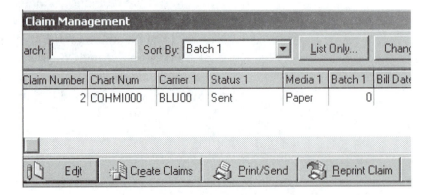

Assume for the purposes of this exercise that the 7.50 payment is received immediately. Apply it to Ms. Cohen's account.

When you finish, your screen should look like this:

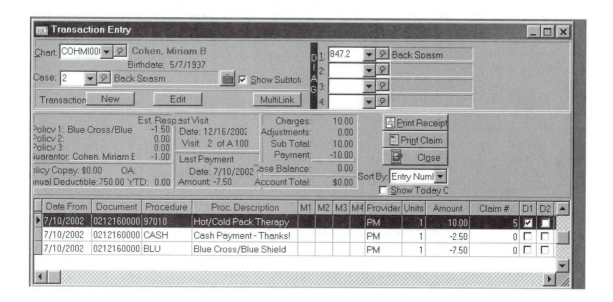

Enter a new case for Karen Wang. Click on the personal tab of the new case dialog box, and fill in the following information:

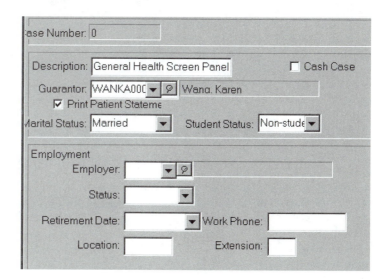

Click on the diagnosis tab and fill in the following information:

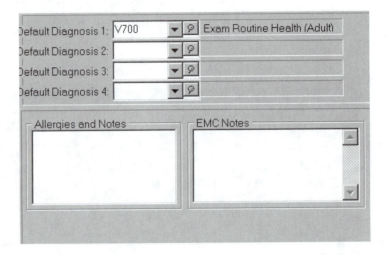

Click on the policy 1 tab and fill in the following information:

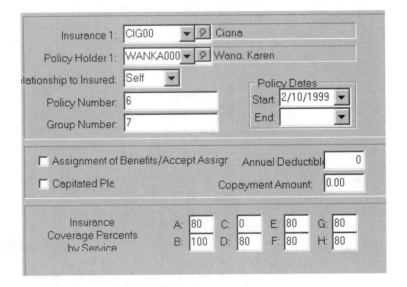

Remember to save the information.

Ms. Wang has an appointment for an exam routine health screen for which the charge is 45.00. Karen has insurance that pays 35.00. Create a claim for Karen Wang. Assume for the purpose of this exercise that Cigna sends the 35.00 immediately. Apply the 35.00 to Ms. Wang's account. The 10.00 is written off by the practice and is an adjustment to Karen's account. To enter transactions for Karen Wang, pull down the activities menu and select enter transactions. You are entering three transactions: one for the charge of 45.00, a second for the Cigna payment of 35.00, and a third for the Cigna write-off of 10.00.

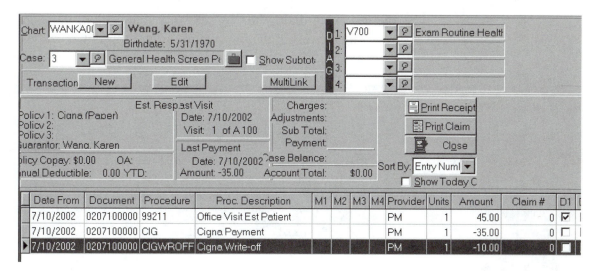

To review, a claim is a bill sent to an insurance carrier. Claim management involves editing, sorting, and sending out claims on paper or electronically.

You have created claims for Miriam Cohen and Karen Wang. You can see the status of all the claims by pulling down the activities menu and selecting claim management. Claims are organized in groups called batches on the basis of the date the claims were created, e.g., all claims created at the same time are in the same batch.

NEW STYLE TRANSACTION ENTRY

In Version 7 Advanced and in Version 8, cases can be created and charges, payments, and adjustments (transactions) entered in one two-paned window. In Version 7 Advanced, pull down the file menu and select program options, click data entry, and click off use old-style transaction. Click save. To enter Joan Q. Adams's case information, including her strep throat diagnosis and procedure, fill in the top of the following dialog box by selecting Joan's chart number, and then selecting the rest of the information from drop-down list boxes:

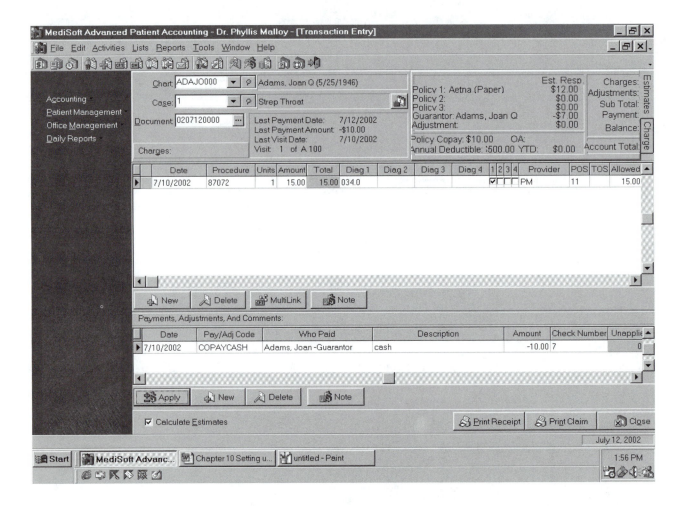

Fill in the payment information in the bottom part of the window. Remember to click the apply command button. Create and send the claim to her insurance.

You can check the status of all your claims in the claim management window. If the list were too long and included claims that were no longer needed, you could delete claims in this window.

PRINTING REPORTS

Every morning the practice prints out a superbill (encounter form) for each patient with an appointment. Make an appointment for Joan Q. Adams for today at 9:00a for a general health screen. Print her superbill by doing the following: Pull down the reports menu and select superbills. In the dialog box that opens, click OK.

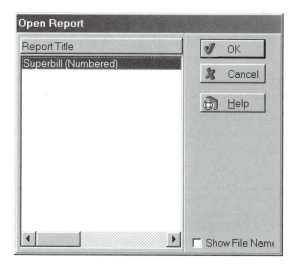

In the print report where? dialog box, click start.

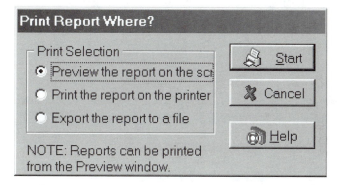

Select Joan Q. Adams's chart number in the chart number range drop-down list boxes in the data selection questions dialog box.

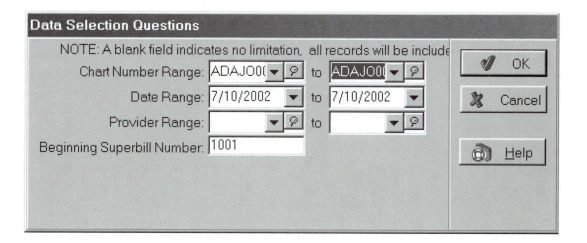

Click OK, and the following superbill will appear:

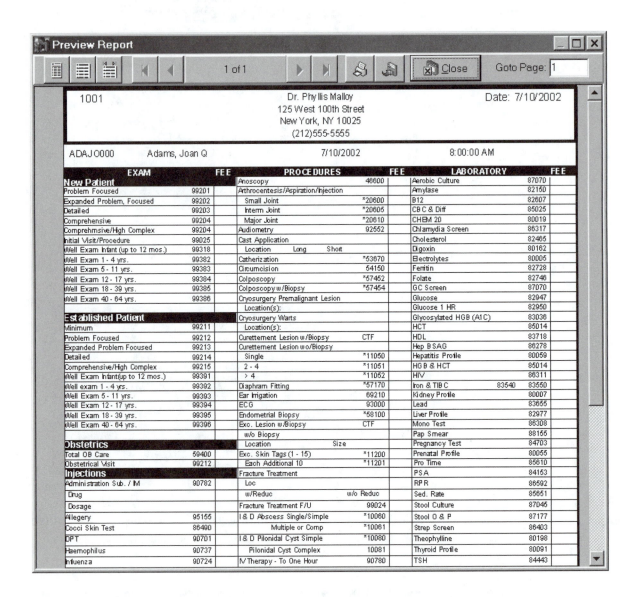

Enter two new transactions for Ms. Adams that reflect the charge of 45.00 and her cash copayment of 10.00. Remember to apply the payment and save the transaction.

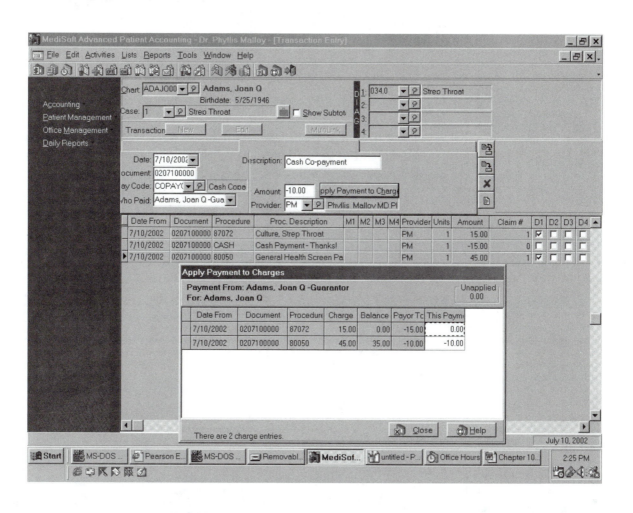

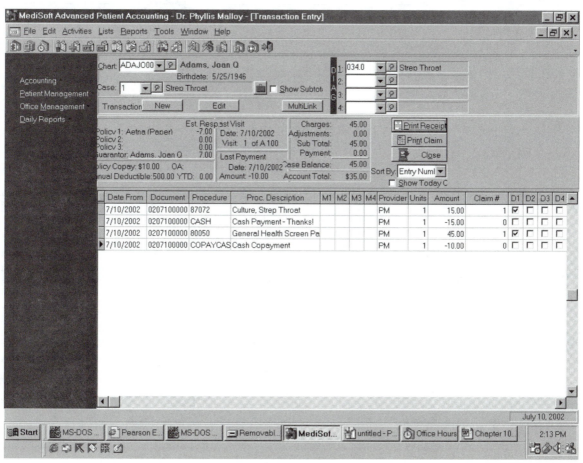

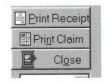

Once the transactions are entered, you can create a walkout receipt to be handed to the patient as he or she is leaving the office. To create a walkout receipt, click print receipt. In the open report dialog box, select walkout receipt (all transactions), and click OK. In the print where? dialog box, click start. In the data selection question dialog box, enter the date of the office visit, and click OK. The following will appear:

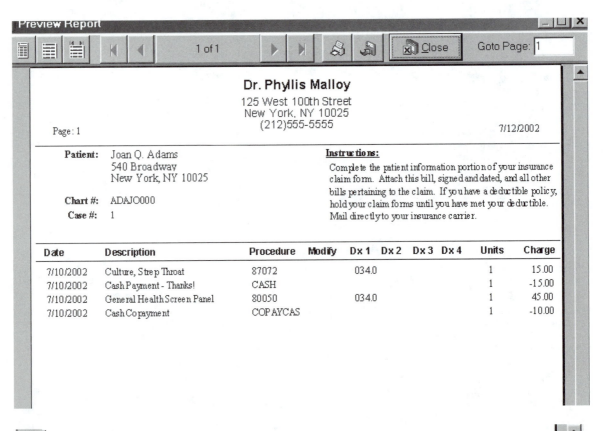

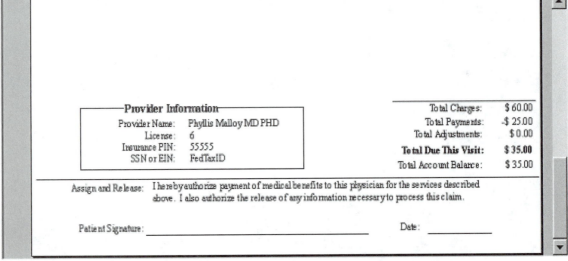

To create a new insurance claim (the bill sent to the insurance carrier), click the print claim command button. Select Joan Q. Adams's chart number.

To print a patient statement for Ms. Adams, pull down the reports menu and select patient statements. Click OK. Click start. Select Joan Q. Adams's chart number in the drop-down list boxes and click OK. The following statement will appear:

Last Payment Received: 7/10/2002	Amount: -10.00		Previous Balance:	0.00
Patient: Joan Q. Adams	Chart #: ADAJO000	Case Description: Strep Throat		
7/10/2002 0207100000	Culture, Strep Throat	1		15.00
7/10/2002 0207100000	Cash Payment - Thanks!	1		-15.00
7/10/2002 0207100000	General Health Screen Panel	1		45.00
7/10/2002 0207100000	Cash Copayment	1		-10.00

Past Due 30 Days	Past Due 60 Days	Past Due 90 Days	Balance Due
0.00	0.00	0.00	**35.00**

A patient day sheet is a report that lists each patient's name, chart number, and transactions for a particular day. To print a patient day sheet, pull down the reports menu and select day sheets. Choose patient day sheet. Click OK. And click OK again. The following report will be generated.

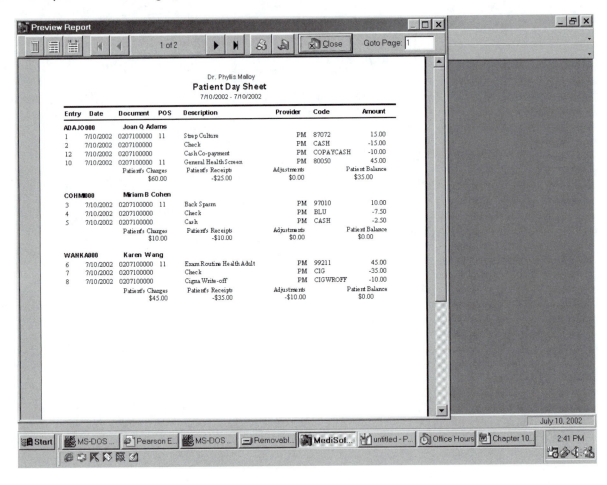

DEPOSIT LIST

To see a **deposit list**, pull down the activities menu and select enter deposits/payments. The following will be displayed:

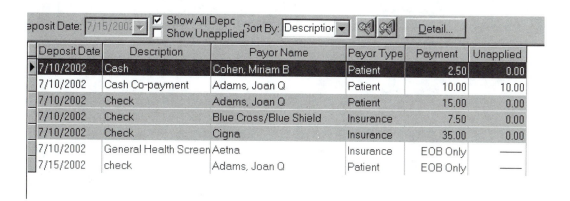

In the deposit list, you can apply payments to charges. Notice that Joan Q. Adams's record has an unapplied payment of 10.00. To apply, select Joan's record and click the apply command button at the bottom of the window. In the apply payment/adjustments to charges dialog box, type 10.00 in the payment box.

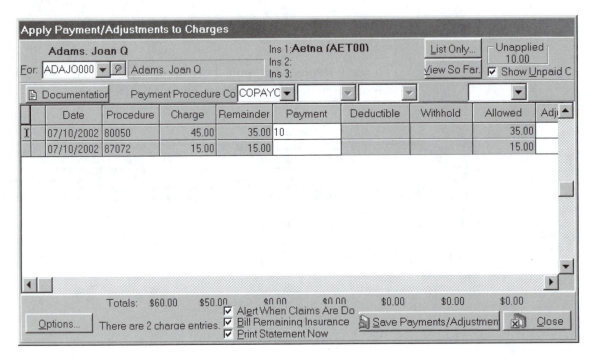

Click the save payments/adjustments command button at the bottom of the window and click close.

The payment is applied:

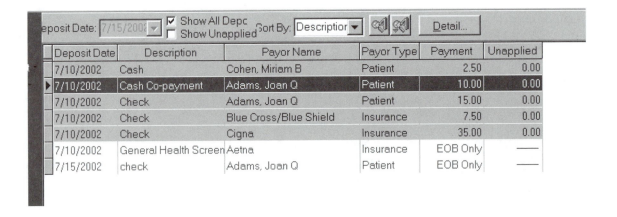

To see a summary of a patient's transactions, click the **quick ledger** button on the toolbar, and select the patient's chart number.

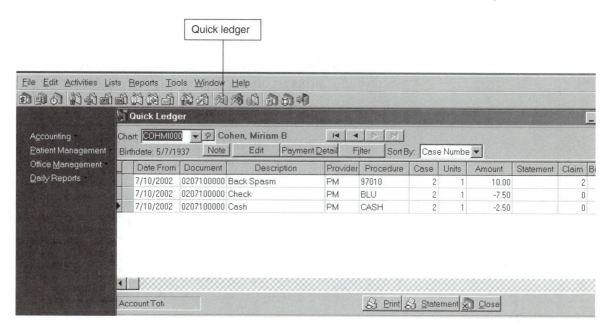

Quick ledger

Click the close command button.

For a summary of a patient's remainder charge totals, click the **quick balance** icon on the toolbar and select the patient's chart number.

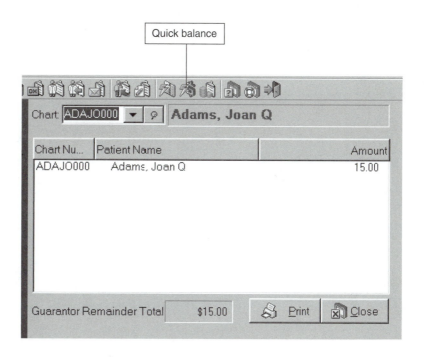

Quick balance

Click close.

Chapter Summary

- MediSoft allows the office worker in a health care environment to enter the information needed to establish a database for a new practice. This includes practice, provider, insurance, address, and diagnosis information.
- Diagnosis codes, billing codes, and procedure, payment, and adjustment codes can also be entered in tables.
- MediSoft is primarily an accounting program. Transactions (charges, payments, and adjustments) can be entered, and payments applied. Claims can be created and sent to insurance carriers.
- Several reports can be generated, including a superbill (encounter form), patient statements, and patient day sheets.
- The deposit list shows the current financial status of patients.

11

Utilities

THIS CHAPTER IS FOR INFORMATION ONLY. YOU <u>CANNOT</u> USE MEDISOFT'S FILE MAINTENANCE AND BACKUP UTILITIES IN A CLASSROOM SETTING.

Chapter Outline

- Learning Objectives
- File Maintenance
- Backup Utility

Learning Objectives

This chapter is for information only. After reading this chapter, the student will be aware of MediSoft's file maintenance and backup utilities.

☐ *FILE MAINTENANCE*

If you were in a working environment and wanted to access Medi-Soft's utility programs, you would pull down the file menu, and choose file maintenance.

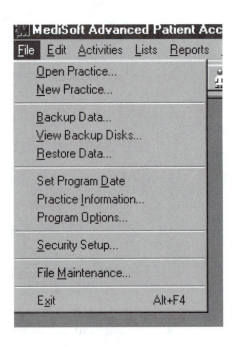

The following screen is displayed:

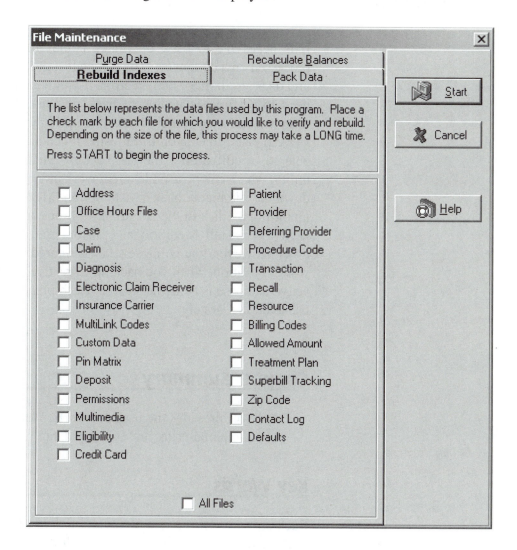

Rebuilding indexes checks the structure of records; it does not change or delete any data.

Packing data compresses data. MediSoft keeps the record structure even after its contents have been deleted. Packing data gets rid of the empty records.

Purging data permanently deletes patients who no longer use the practice. It can also be used to delete cases, appointments, claims, and audit data. Extreme care should be used.

Recalculating balances updates balances, so that they reflect the newest entries.

BACKUP UTILITY

It is necessary to back up (make copies of files on disk) all data processed on a computer. Data can be lost due to computer failure, natural disaster, theft, or human error. If you were in an office, you would need to set up a schedule to back up your data. Daily backups to diskettes and then weekly backups to a higher capacity medium such as a zip disk protect you from losing much data; you only lose what is entered or edited after the last backup. MediSoft provides a backup utility, which can be used in a real work environment; to access it, pull down the file menu, backup data option. MediSoft data can be backed up on floppy disk in the A:\ drive. If your computer crashes, you may need to reinstall MediSoft and restore the data using your backup disks. However, you will lose all data entered after your last backup. A word of caution, when you back up a practice's database files, only the active database is being backed up. Each practice's database should be backed up separately.

Chapter Summary

- MediSoft provides the user in an office environment with utilities to help maintain files and back up data.

Key Words

Back up   Rebuilding indexes
Packing data   Recalculating balances
Purging data

REVIEW EXERCISES

1. Define the following terms:

   Packing data

   Purging data

   Rebuilding indexes

   Recalculating balances

2. Discuss why it is necessary to back up your data on disk. In your answer, refer to the various threats to computer systems and data.

Addendum

New in Version 8

The MediSoft Version 8 toolbars and icons are essentially the same as those in Version 7.

The MediSoft Version 8 Toolbar

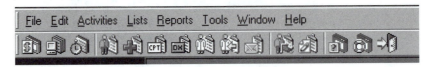

MediSoft Office Hours Toolbar Version 8

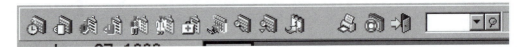

There are several new features in MediSoft Version 8:

- There are fields for emergency contacts and cell phone numbers in the patient/guarantor, provider, and address windows.
- Transaction entry is done in a single two-paned window, similar to the new style transaction entry in Version 7. Version 8 can process credit card transactions.
- The user can set the program to hyphenate Social Security numbers automatically, by pulling down the file menu, choosing program options, selecting data entry, and clicking on Social Security number.

There are additional changes in MediSoft Advanced Professional:

- Printing can be done from almost any window using the print grid button or the right-click menu.
- The ability to search has been expanded.
- Quick receipts can be printed from the transaction entry window and quick statements from the quick ledger window.

Appendix

1

Introduction to Computers and Computer Literacy

Outline

- Computer Literacy
- What Is a Computer?
- Data Representation
- Computer Hardware
  - Input Devices
  - Processing Hardware and Memory
  - Output Devices
  - Secondary Storage Devices
- Software
  - Systems Software
  - Applications Software
- The Data Processing Cycle
- Appendix Summary
- Key Words
- Further Reading

Learning Objectives

Upon completion of this appendix, the student will be able to:

- Define the terms computer literacy and computer
- Discuss how the computer represents data
- Define computer hardware and software
- Comprehend the data processing cycle

COMPUTER LITERACY

A general knowledge of computers, their uses in any career or field, particularly health care is essential.

Computer literacy refers to knowledge of how to use computer information technology. The details of the definition of computer literacy are continually changing as computers and their uses change. Currently, computer literacy involves several aspects. A computer literate person knows how to use a computer in his or her own field to make tasks easier and to complete them more efficiently, has a vocabulary to discuss computers intelligently, and understands in a broad general fashion what a computer is and what it can do. Today, unlike several years ago, computer literacy involves knowledge of the **Internet** and the **World Wide Web** and the ability to take advantage of these resources. Being computer literate does not mean you can build, fix, or program a computer. Familiarity with computers and the Internet is crucial in any field, including health care and its delivery. As in other fields, the basic tasks of gathering, allocating, controlling, and retrieving information are the same.

In the year 2003, very few people question the necessity of learning about computers, although some are afraid of the new technology. Knowledge is the best way to overcome this anxiety. It is definitely worth making the effort, since, in every discipline, computers are playing a larger and more important role, and almost any employed person will have to be a competent computer **user**. This is particularly true in the field of health care and medical office management, where the ability to learn to use new programs specifically geared to medical office management can mean the difference between employment and unemployment.

WHAT IS A COMPUTER?

A **computer** is an electronic device that can accept **data** (raw facts) as input, and process, manipulate, or alter them in some way, and produce useful **information** as output. A computer processes data by following step-by-step instructions called a program. The program, the data, and the information need to be stored temporarily in memory while processing is going on, and permanently on a secondary storage device for future use. Computers are accurate, fast, and reliable. Computers can be classified according to their size and power. However, every computer performs similar functions.

Classification of Computers by Size and Power

Supercomputer	Is the fastest, most powerful computer available at any time. Supercomputers are used for scientific purposes—to simulate actual events so that prediction is possible. Supercomputers are used to forecast the weather, to simulate events such as a car crash, to simulate the structure of a virus on the screen.
Mainframe	Is smaller than a supercomputer. A mainframe is a multiuser system with many terminals using the power of one computer in what is called a timesharing environment. Unlike the supercomputer, the mainframe is used for business purposes, for repetitive tasks such as generating a payroll or processing insurance claims.
Microcomputer or Personal Computer (PC)	Is a single-user computer. Microcomputers come in different sizes, from a small notebook to a powerful workstation. Microcomputers can be networked, making the information and programs available on one PC available to all on the network. When linked to the Internet, a microcomputer puts the world at your fingertips.
Embedded Computer	Is a microprocessor that does one thing, such as regulate a heart pacemaker. It is embedded in the appliance, and can be programmed to respond to changing conditions, for example, to help the heart when help is needed.

Computer hardware includes all of the physical components of a computer. Each computer function that is performed has hardware associated with it: **Input devices** for entering data which we as people understand and converting it into a form that the computer can process; a **processing unit** for manipulating data; **output devices** to produce information useful to human beings; memory for temporary storage; and secondary storage devices for more permanent storage.

DATA REPRESENTATION

All data in a computer is represented by bits (binary digits). This includes characters, numbers, graphics, sound, animation, and so on. A bit is either a one or a zero.

☐ COMPUTER HARDWARE

Input Devices   Input hardware functions to enter data that you understand and digitize it or translate it into a form that the computer can process, that is, zeros and ones, offs and ons. Input devices can be divided into **keyboards** and **direct-entry devices**.

Keyboards

The keyboard with which you are familiar is called the **QWERTY** keyboard. It was invented during the nineteenth century for the mechanical typewriter. The arrangement of the keys was meant to slow typists down, because if they typed too fast, the keys would jam. The keyboard most of us use is not conducive to fast data entry. It can also contribute to **carpal tunnel syndrome**, which is a painful compression of the median nerve in the wrist and the hand caused by repetitive motion. The field of **ergonomics** attempts to study the relationship between people and their work environment and to minimize work-related injuries and to create a safer and more efficient workplace.

The standard QWERTY keyboard contains several kinds of keys: the **alphanumeric** keyboard (letters and numbers) and special symbol keys (such as @, &, *, etc.). The enter key is used to end a paragraph and enter commands; special **function keys** perform different tasks depending on the software you are using. When you press any key on the keyboard, it is immediately translated into machine language, a series of electronic pulses that the computer can process.

Direct-Entry Devices

Direct-entry devices include **pointing devices** (such as a mouse, trackball, touch screen, and various kinds of pen-based input). **Pen-based systems** recognize handwriting. They are used in some hospitals to enter comments on a patient's chart. **Scanning devices** translate images into digital form by shining light on the image and measuring the reflection. Scanning devices include the bar-code scanner found in every supermarket; **optical mark recognition (OMR)**, which can sense a mark by a number 2 pencil on a Scantron sheet; **optical character recognition (OCR),** which reads printed characters; and the **Kurzweil scanner**, which reads printed material aloud and is useful to those with impaired vision.

An early scanning device used in the banking industry reads the numbers printed on checks in magnetic ink. **Magnetic ink character recognition (MICR)** recognizes a small character set, and is used almost exclusively by banks.

A **fax machine** is also a scanning device. It scans the text or image and converts it to electronic signals that are sent over phone lines; the receiving fax machine converts it back into text and images. A fax machine can scan whole pages of graphics and text and digitize them so that the computer can process them. Once scanned in, you can treat the text in the same way as text you typed in.

Various types of cards are also used as input devices. The **magnetic stripe** on the back of your charge card or ATM card contains data, for example, your account number, in a form a computer can read. A **smart card** looks like other cards, but contains a microprocessor chip and memory. It can do some processing and hold about thirty pages worth of data. Smart cards are used as debit cards. An **optical card** holds about 2,000 pages of data. An optical card could be used to hold your whole medical history, including test results and X rays. Small enough to carry in your wallet, the information on the optical card would be immediately available if you were hospitalized in an emergency.

Speech input systems began as adaptive technology to help people with vision impairments and people who could not use a keyboard. They allow the user to talk to the computer; the computer will then digitize the spoken words. A speech recognition system contains a dictionary of digital patterns of words. You say a word, and the system digitizes it and compares it to the words in its dictionary. Speech recognition systems have to be trained to recognize your speech; the more you talk to it, the more it understands your speech.

A computer uses a **digital camera** to digitize images and stores the images. The computer sees by having the camera take a picture of an object. The digitized image of this object is then compared with the images in storage. This may be used to develop special glasses for Alzheimer patients that can identify people and attach a name to the face.

Of particular interest to health professionals are input devices called sensors. A **sensor** is a device that collects data directly from the environment and sends the data to a computer. Sensors are used to collect patient information for clinical monitoring systems, including physiological, arrhythmia, pulmonary, and obstetrical/neonatal systems. They can detect the smallest change in temperature or any other physiological measurement.

The newest kinds of input devices allow you to use your body as an input device. Biometrics are being used in security systems to protect data from unauthorized users. Fingerprints, handprints, and iris scans are being used to identify authorized users. Human biology input devices include line-of-sight and brain wave input. With **line-of-sight systems**, the user's eyes can point to a part of the screen; a camera and computer can identify the area where you are looking. Line-of-sight input can be used by people who do not have the use of their limbs. If the user looks at a letter for a certain amount of time, it is as if she or he typed that letter on the keyboard. Brain wave input involves implanting a chip in a locked-in stroke victim; this has been successfully done, and has allowed people who could not communicate to write sentences on a computer screen by thinking!

Processing Hardware and Memory

Once data are input into the computer, they are processed—manipulated in some way. Located on the main circuit board (**motherboard**), the **processor** or **system unit** contains the **central processing unit (CPU)** and **memory**. In a microcomputer the microprocessor is on a chip. In a larger computer, the processor might be on several circuit boards. The CPU has two parts. The **arithmetic-logic unit (ALU)** performs the arithmetic operations of adding, subtracting, multiplying, dividing, and raising to a power, as well as the logical operation of comparing. The **control unit (CU)** directs the operation of the computer in accordance with the program's instructions.

The CPU works closely with memory—the computer's temporary workspace. The instructions of the program being executed must be in memory for processing to take place. Memory is also located on the computer's main circuit board. The central processing unit fetches one instruction at a time from memory and processes it.

The part of memory where current work is temporarily stored during processing is called **random access memory (RAM)**. RAM is also on chips. It is temporary, volatile memory. Its contents disappear when the power is turned off. The size of RAM is important, since the program you are executing and the work you create must be able to fit in RAM. Remember, that a **byte** is eight bits—about the space it takes to store one character.

The Capacity of RAM Is Measured In

Kilobyte	(K, Kb)	is approximately one thousand bytes
Megabyte	(M, Mb)	is approximately one million bytes
Gigabyte	(G, Gb)	is approximately one billion bytes
Terabyte	(T, Tb)	is approximately one trillion bytes
Petabyte	(P, Pb)	is approximately one quadrillion bytes or 1,048,576 gigabytes

A small part of RAM is called **cache** memory; it is a special high-speed temporary storage area that holds the most often-used instructions. Data and instructions are moved from cache memory or RAM to the CPU on electronic pathways called **buses**. The other part of memory (also on chips) is called **read only memory (ROM)** or firmware. ROM is permanent and contains basic start-up instructions for the computer; you cannot change the contents of ROM.

Several factors determine the speed of a computer, including the size of RAM, word size, and clock speed. The size of RAM affects the speed of the computer. If RAM is not big enough to hold what you are working with, your work is slowed considerably. Computer processors are made to handle a certain number of bits as a unit at one time. This is called its **word size**. The bigger the word size, the faster the processor. Processors contain a **system clock**, a vibrating quartz crystal. The speed of the vibrations controls the speed of the processor. In a PC, clock speed is measured in **megahertz** (MHz; 1 million cycles per second).

Output Devices

Once data are processed, output devices translate what the computer understands (bits) into a form human beings understand. Output devices are divided into two basic categories: those that produce **hard copy** such as **printers** and **plotters**; and those that produce **soft copy** such as **monitors** and **speech output systems**.

Printers may be **impact** printers, where a print head actually strikes the paper, or **nonimpact**. **Dot-matrix printers** are impact printers that form characters with pins in the shape of the character striking an inked ribbon. Inexpensive and noisy, dot-matrix printers do not produce excellent output. Today, nonimpact printers are more common. **Ink-jet printers** form letters by spraying dots of ink on paper. Ink-jet printers produce excellent quality text and graphics in black and white and color at a low cost. **Laser printers** produce the best output, but are the most expensive. The technology used by laser printers is similar to that used by Xerox machines. For specialized graphics output, plotters can be used. Plotters are used to create maps and architectural drawings.

The most commonly used output device is a monitor. Screens differ in size, color, and in the clarity of the display. Soft copy is also produced by devices that output sound, music, and speech.

Secondary Storage Devices

The memory we have discussed so far is temporary or volatile. In order to **save** your work more permanently, you need secondary storage devices. **Magnetic disk** (**diskette** or **hard disk**), **magnetic tape**, and **optical disks** are used as secondary storage media. Magnetic media store data and programs as magnetic spots or electromagnetic charges. Optical disks store data as pits and lands burnt into a plastic disk.

To use a diskette, it is inserted into a **secondary storage device** such as a **disk drive**, which has a motor to spin the disk and an access arm with a **read/write head** to move across it. It is this read/write head that reads data from (makes a copy of the data to put in RAM) and writes data to (takes what is in RAM and puts it on the disk) the diskette. A hard disk is similar, but includes several platters made of metal or glass, and is encased in a sealed unit to keep contaminants away from the disk surfaces. Data are recorded on both sides of the platters. Hard disks hold much more data than floppies—up to several gigabytes. Access time is much faster; they spin continuously at a much higher rate of speed. A potential disadvantage of hard drives is the possibility of a **head crash**; the cushion of air between the read/write head and the disk is tiny and the disk is spinning so fast that any contamination can cause the head to touch the disk and may destroy the data.

Optical disks use laser technology to store data as pits and lands (flat areas) on a disk. Instead of an access arm and read/write head, a high-power laser burns tiny pits in the surface, and another lower-power laser reads the surface, interpreting the pits and lands as zeroes and ones. The pits are so small that an enormous amount of data can be stored on one laser disk. Three thousand pits take up only one centimeter.

There are several kinds of optical disk: **CD-ROM (compact disk-read only memory)** is the most common. A CD-ROM is created at a factory; you can buy it, put it in your CD-ROM drive, and read the contents into the memory of your PC. However, you cannot change the contents of the CD-ROM. Their immense storage capacity of 680M is roughly equivalent to 477 high-density 3.5" diskettes, or about 250,000 pages. This volume makes them ideal for distributing books and encyclopedias.

A **CD-R (compact disk-recordable)** is sold as a blank disk on which the user can create his or her own CD-ROM. Once created, however, it cannot be changed. A **CD-RW (compact disk rewriteable)** can be read from and written to—much like a diskette. **DVD** disks (digital video or digital versatile disks) are optical disks with a storage capacity of 4.7 gigabytes. A super DVD can hold up to 17 gigabytes.

Some of the advantages of optical disks include their great capacity, low cost, and durability. An optical disk lasts longer than magnetic media.

The oldest form of secondary storage is magnetic tape. The difference between retrieving data from tape and disk of any kind is like the difference between listening to music on audiotape and compact disk. A disk allows **direct access** to any piece of information on that specific disk. Unlike a disk, a tape is a **sequential access storage medium**. To get to the 500th piece of information on tape, you need to fast forward through the first 499, in the same way as you would listen to the third song on an audiotape, that is, you have to fast forward through the first two. A tape cartridge is loaded into a drive where the tape passes under a read/write head. Magnetic tape comes in different widths and lengths. It is the slowest and cheapest medium, but holds a great deal of data. Today it is used mainly for backing up disk storage.

Larger computers use hard disks for secondary storage. The disks differ in the size of the platters, the number of platters, and the recording capacity.

SOFTWARE

Software refers to the programs, that is, the step-by-step instructions that tell the hardware what to do. Without software, hardware is useless. Software falls into two general categories: system software and applications software.

System Software

System software consists of programs that help the computer manage its own resources. The most important piece of system software is the operating system. The operating system is a group of programs that manages the resources of the computer. It controls the hardware, manages basic input and output operations, keeps track of files saved on disk and in memory, and directs communication between the CPU and other pieces of hardware. It coordinates how other programs work with the hardware and with each other. Operating systems also provide the **user interface**, that is, the way the user communicates with the computer. For example, Windows provides a **graphical user interface**, pictures or icons that you click on with a mouse. When the computer is turned on, the operating system is booted or loaded into the computer's RAM. No other program can work until the operating system is booted. There are several operating systems for microcomputers, including DOS (disk operating system), Windows 95/98/2000/XP, UNIX, and Macintosh. Utility programs such as screen savers and backup software are also examples of system software.

Applications Software

Applications software allows you to apply computer technology to a task you need done. There are applications packages for many needs.

Word processing software allows you to enter text for a paper, report, letter, or memo. Once it is entered, it can be edited (corrected and improved) and formatted (changed in appearance). The size, style, and face of the type, margins and justification, line spacing, and tab stops can all be changed.

Electronic spreadsheets allow you to process numerical data. Organized into rows and columns intersecting to form cells, spreadsheets make doing arithmetic almost fun. You enter the values you want processed and the formula that tells the software how to process the values, and the answer appears. If you find you made a mistake entering a value, just change it, and the answer is **automatically recalculated**. Spreadsheet software also allows the creation of graphs. Spreadsheets have several health care related applications. The Food and Drug Administration uses giant spreadsheets to keep records of clinical trials. A spreadsheet program can help with anything that can be reduced to numbers, such as tracking the spread of a disease, a hospital's financial planning, and materials management.

Database management software (DBMS) allows you to manage large quantities of data in an organized fashion. Information in a database is organized in tables. The database management software makes it easy to enter data, edit it, sort or organize it, search for data that meets a particular criterion, and retrieve the data. Once the structure of the table is defined and the data entered, the data never have to be typed again; attractive reports can be generated easily by simply defining their structure—not retyping the data. **MediSoft** allows the user to create relational databases, which can link tables of doctors, patients, cases, insurance codes, allowed amounts, procedure codes, and diagnostic codes. All this information is necessary to the running of a medical office and the accurate generation of bills.

Appendix Summary

- Computer literacy refers to the ability to use computers in your field, to use the Internet, to be able to discuss computers intelligently.

- A computer is an electronic device that accepts data as input, then processes the data and displays (on screen or paper) information as output. Information, data, and programs can be saved temporarily or permanently. The computer operates under the control of programs stored in memory. All computers perform the four functions of input-process-storage-output.

- Data are represented inside the computer by zeroes and ones, offs and ons.

- Computer hardware refers to the parts of the computer you can see, including input and output devices, processing hardware and internal memory, and secondary storage devices.

- System software includes programs that perform basic functions for the computer. The operating system takes care of basic input and output, keeps track of files, and manages processor time. Applications software does a task for you: Word processing programs allow you to type text documents. Electronic spreadsheets make math quick and easy. Database management software helps you organize huge masses of data.

Key Words

Applications software
Arithmetic-logic unit (ALU)
Automatic recalculation
Binary digit
Bit
Boot
Bus
Byte
Cache
Carpal tunnel syndrome
CD-R (compact disk-recordable)
CD-ROM (compact disk-read only memory)
CD-RW (compact disk rewriteable)
Central processing unit (CPU)
Computer
Computer literacy
Control unit (CU)
Data
Data representation
Database management software (DBMS)
Digital camera
Digitize
Direct access
Direct-entry devices
Disk drive
Diskette
Dot-matrix printer

DVD
Electronic spreadsheet
Embedded computer
Ergonomics
Fax machine
Graphical user interface (GUI)
Hard copy
Hard disk
Hardware
Head crash
Impact printer
Information
Ink-jet printer
Input device
Internet
Keyboard
Kilobyte (K, Kb)
Kurzweil scanner
Laser printer
Line-of-sight system
Magnetic disk
Magnetic ink character recognition (MICR)
Magnetic stripe
Magnetic tape
Mainframe
Megabyte (M, Mb)
Megahertz
Memory
Microcomputer

Monitor
Motherboard
Nonimpact printer
Operating system (OS)
Optical card
Optical character recognition
  (OCR)
Optical disk
Optical mark recognition (OMR)
Output device
Pen-based system
Personal computer (PC)
Petabyte (P, Pb)
Plotter
Pointing device
Printer
Processing hardware
Processing unit
Processor
Program
QWERTY
Random access memory (RAM)
Read only memory (ROM)
Read/write head

Scanning device
Secondary storage device
Secondary storage medium
Sensor
Sequential access storage
  medium
Smart card
Soft copy
Software
Speech input system
Speech output system
Supercomputer
System clock
System software
System unit
Tape
Terabyte (T, Tb)
User
User interface
Utility program
Word processing software
Word size
World Wide Web

Further Reading

Sara Baase. *A Gift of Fire: Social, Legal, and Ethical Issues in Computing.* Upper Saddle River, N.J.: Prentice-Hall, 1996.

Burke, Lillian, and Barbara Weill. *Information Technology for the Health Professions.* Upper Saddle River, N.J.: Brady/Prentice-Hall Health, 2000.

Chase, Victor. "Mind over Muscles." http://www.techreview.com/articles/med00/chase . . . htm (March/April 2000: February 22, 2000), 6 pages.

"A Computer 'Reads' Minds." http://abcnews.go.com/sections/science/DailyNews/computer_readmind000113.html, 1 page.

Hyde, Joe. "Report: Computer ownership is up but 'digital divide' persists," wysiwyg/:51/http://www.ada.org/prof/pubs/daily/netnews/stories/divide.html (April 20, 2001; July 12, 2001), 2 pages.

Meyer, Marilyn, and Roberta Baber. *Computers in Your Future.* Indianapolis, Ind.: Que E & T, 1997.

Nagourney, Eris. "Visiting the Doctor via the Dining Room." NYT.com (April 6, 1999; April 8, 1999).

Oakman, Robert. *The Computer Triangle,* 2d ed. New York: John Wiley and Sons, 1997.

O'Neil, John. "In Future, Some Doctors May Be Gadgets." NYT.com (May 18, 1999; July 12, 2001), 5 pages.

Glossary

Accounts Receivable (A/R)   any invoices or payments from the patient or insurance carriers to the medical practice

ADAM   a computer simulation program that teaches anatomy using text and graphics

Adjustment   a positive or negative change to a patient account

Administrative application   computer application that includes office management, scheduling, and billing tasks

Aging reports   reflect amounts owed or claims filed by age

Allowed amount   each insurance carrier allows a certain amount for each procedure performed; the allowed amount helps determine what the insurance company pays

Analysis reports   there are several kinds of analysis reports including practice analysis and insurance analysis reports

Applications software   software such as word processors, spreadsheets, and DBMS that apply computer technology to a task you need done

Appointment grid   a day's or week's appointments on a calendar grid

Appointment list   a list of appointments for a day which can be printed

Arithmetic-logic unit (ALU)   the part of the central processing unit that does arithmetic and performs logical operations

Arrow   mouse pointer shape; used to point

Assigned provider   the health care provider that a particular patient uses

Assignment   the amount the insurance company pays for a procedure and a provider agrees to accept

Audit/edit report   if your office uses a clearinghouse to process electronic claims, it utilizes an audit/edit report to see whether all the necessary information is included and accurate; used by offices that use a clearinghouse to process electronic claims

Authorization   permission by the insurance carrier for the provider to perform a medical procedure

Automatic recalculation   if the user changes a value in a cell in an electronic spreadsheet, and a formula refers to that cell, the computer calculates the answer again to reflect the change the user made

Back up   to copy files and data onto a secondary storage medium

Balance billing (bucket billing)   system used in health care environments in which the first insurer is billed; when it responds, the EOB (explanation of benefits) and bill are sent to the secondary insurer; when it responds, the EOBs and bill are sent to the tertiary insurer; and only when all insurers have responded is a bill sent to the patient or guarantor.

Batch   claims are organized in groups called batches, depending on the date of their creation

Billing code   groups patients for billing purposes

Billing/payment status report   report that shows current billing, payment, and claim status of each transaction.

Binary digit (bit)   1 or 0

Biometrics (biometric method)   security measure; uses an aspect of the authorized user's body to identify her or him; includes fingerprints, handprints, iris scans, etc.

Bit (binary digit)   1 or 0

Boot   load the operating system into memory

Bucket billing (balance billing)   billing system used in health care environments in which the first insurer is billed; when it responds, the EOB and bill are sent to the secondary insurer; when it responds, the EOBs and bill are sent to the tertiary insurer; and only when all insurers have responded is a bill sent to the patient or guarantor

Bus   an electronic pathway along which data travels within the computer during processing

Byte   eight bits; the space it takes to store one character in memory

Cache   a form of memory that holds the most frequently used data and instructions; its purpose is to speed processing

Callback system   a security system for networks whereby a user calls in to the computer, hangs up, and the computer calls back to one authorized phone

Capitated plan   insurance plan in which a physician is paid a fixed fee (the capitation), and the physician is paid regardless of the amount of treatment he or she provides. Some patients may seek no treatment; some may visit several times

Carpal tunnel syndrome   a repetitive stress injury; involves the painful compression of the nerves in the wrist and hand

Case   the condition for which the patient visits the doctor

Case billing code   groups cases, e.g., the case billing code for Medicare patients is M

Case number   the number a case is assigned; case numbers are assigned by MediSoft

CD-R (compact disk-recordable)   an optical device; a secondary storage medium on which data are represented by pits and lands; can be written to and read from

CD-ROM (compact disk-read only memory)   optical device; secondary storage medium on which data are stored as pits and lands; created and read by lasers; the user can read from but not write to this medium

CD-RW (compact disk rewriteable)   optical device on which the user can read and write data; secondary storage medium on which data are stored as pits and lands; created and read by lasers

Center for Medicaid and State Operations (CMS)   new name for Health Care Financing Administration (HCFA)

Central processing unit (CPU)   the "brains" of the computer; comprised of the control unit and the arithmetic-logic unit

CHAMPVA   a federal health benefits program that supplements medical care in the military

Charge   the amount a patient is billed for the provider's service

Chart number   consists of the first three letters of the patient's last name, the first two letters of the first name, and three additional digits; the chart number is assigned by MediSoft

Check box   an element of a dialog box; one (or none) or more choices can be made from a set of check boxes

Claim   a request to an insurance company for payment for services

Claim management   includes all tasks involved in creating, submitting, sending, printing claims

Claim summary   report that lists the status of claims

Clearinghouse   a business that collects insurance claims from providers and sends them to the correct insurance carrier

Click   basic mouse operation in which the user presses the left mouse button and releases it

Clinical application   computer application which is involved in direct patient care; includes diagnostic tools, and medical monitoring devices

Close button   button that closes windows or applications

CMS   Center for Medicaid and State Operations (new name for HCFA)

Command button   an element of a dialog box used to enter a command such as OK or cancel

Computer   an electronic device that—under the control of a stored program—accepts data as input, processes it, produces information as output, and may store the results.

Computer literacy   general knowledge of computers and the Internet, and the ability to use computers in your own field or profession

Computerized tomography (CT) scan   imaging technique in which a computer produces a 2- or 3-dimensional picture by using a formula to combine the information of many X rays

Condition   the reason that a patient seeks treatment from a health care provider

Connectivity   the fact that computers can be linked to each other to form a network

Control unit (CU)   hardware that controls processing; part of the central processing unit (CPU)

Copayment   under managed care, the patient may be required to pay a small copayment to a participating provider

CPT (Current Procedural Terminology)   services including tests, lab work, exams, and treatments are coded using CPTs (*Current Procedural Terminology*, 4th ed.)

Custom report   a report whose structure is designed by the user

Custom report grid   grid on which the user designs a report structure

Data   raw facts that are input to the computer to be processed

Data audit report   report that lists any changes or deletions made in transaction

Data field   a field in a report that takes data from the tables the user has entered

Data representation   a computer represents all data using binary digits (bits)

Database   an organized collection of data

Database management software (DBMS)   software that allows the user to create, access, organize and reorganize, and maintain an organized collection of related data

Day sheets   include patient, procedure, and payment day sheets

Decryption   unscrambling of encrypted data; only an authorized user has the decryption software

Deductible   a certain amount the patient is required to pay each year before the insurance begins paying

Deposit list   lists payments, their source and type, description, and whether or not the payment has been applied

Desktop   the screen on the monitor on which Windows displays icons representing hardware and programs

Detail lines   the lines on a report that change from record to record, taking each patient's information from the original tables

Dialog box   a window used for collecting information

Digital camera   a camera that digitizes and stores images

Direct access   any form of disk storage (hard disk, diskette, optical disk); allows the read/write head or laser to go directly to any piece of data

Direct-entry device   input devices including pointing and drawing devices and scanning devices

Disk drive   storage device; a diskette is inserted into the drive which spins; an access arm with a read/write head moves over the disk and reads from or writes to the disk

Diskette   secondary storage medium

Dot-matrix printer   an impact printer that creates hard copy using a printhead made up of pins striking an inked ribbon, which then hits the paper

Double-click   a basic mouse operation in which the user clicks the left mouse button twice

Drag   a basic mouse operation in which the user holds down the left mouse button while moving the mouse

DRG (diagnosis related group)   coding systems include DRG (diagnosis related group); hospital reimbursement by private and government insurers is determined by diagnosis; each patient is given a DRG classification, and a formula based on this classification determines reimbursement

Drop-down list box   element of a dialog box that allows the user to choose an option by clicking on a down arrow to access the choices and selecting one by clicking on it with the mouse

Electronic appointment book   MediSoft's appointment scheduler

Electronic claim management   insurance claim submission over telecommunications lines

Electronic funds transfer (EFT)   the electronic transfer of funds used to pay an electronic media claim; the funds transfer can be accompanied by an electronic remittance advice (ERA) explaining the response to the claim

Electronic media claim (EMC)   claim submitted to insurance carriers electronically

Electronic medical record (EMR)   a patient's complete medical history (including tests, notes, vaccinations, etc.) in electronic form; should include dental records, and the records of all the other health care providers the patient has consulted

Electronic remittance advice (ERA)   accompanies the response to an EMC (electronic media claim); explanation from the insurance company of why certain services were covered and others not

Electronic spreadsheets   applications software that allows the user to work with math

Embedded computer   a single-purpose computer on a chip; embedded in appliances from a toaster or wristwatch to a pacemaker

Encounter form (superbill)   a list of diagnoses and procedures common to the practice

Encryption   a security measure that attempts to safeguard data by scrambling it; only authorized personnel have the decryption software

Ergonomics   the study of the relationship of the work environment to the worker's health

Expert system   software that turns the computer into an expert in a specific field; the computer is fed facts and rules about how the facts are used in decision making; some expert systems in health care are mycin, internist, POEMS, and PKC (problem knowledge coupler)

Explanation of benefits (EOB)   explanation from the insurance company of why certain services were covered and others not

Fax machine   a scanning device that transmits text and graphics via telecommunications lines

Fee-for-service plans   using a fee-for-service plan, the patient is never restricted to a network of providers and needs no referrals for specialists. After fulfilling a deductible (a certain amount the patient is required to pay each year before the insurance begins paying), every visit to a doctor is paid for by the insurance company

Field   one piece of information in a record in a database table

File   a collection of data stored on disk; within any MediSoft database, there is a separate file for patients, doctors, insurance companies, etc.

File maintenance   MediSoft utilities for backing up data, rebuilding indexes, purging data, and re-calculating balances allow the user to keep files up to date and complete

File menu   contains options that allow the user to open an existing database for a practice or establish a new database for a new practice

Filter   reports can be filtered to select a particular date range and a particular patient or patients

Firewall   an attempt to protect private networks using an electronic block

Footer   information across the bottom of a page in a report

Formatting toolbar   toolbar on which the user can find buttons to format text, such as the bold, italic, underline, and alignment buttons, etc.

Function help line   shortcut bar

Function keys   keys whose function changes according to the software used

Gigabyte (G, Gb)   about 1 billion bytes

Global commands   commands that function anywhere in a program to do the same thing

Graphical user interface (GUI)   user interface in which the user communicates with the computer by using a mouse to click on icons

Guarantor   the person who is responsible for paying the bill

Hand   a basic mouse pointer shape; the mouse pointer is a hand when choosing help topics

Hard copy   output on paper; produced by printers and plotters

Hard disk   secondary storage device in which several platters of metal or ceramic spin at a high rate of speed; read/write heads on access arms can read from or write to all surfaces of the disks; higher capacity, faster, and more reliable than diskette

Hardware   the physical components of a computer

HCFA   Health Care Financing Administration (recently changed to CMS)

HCFA-1500   most commonly used and accepted claim form

Head crash   any contamination that gets into a hard drive can cause the read/write head to come into contact with the disk and damage the disk and information on it

Header   information across the top of a report

Health Care Financing Administration (HCFA)   the agency that administers government-funded health care insurance plans (see CMS)

Health Insurance Portability and Accountability Act of 1996 (see HIPAA)   the first federal legislation dealing with the privacy of medical information

Health maintenance organization (HMO)   patient who uses a health maintenance organization (HMO) pays a fixed yearly fee, and must choose among an approved network of health care providers and hospitals; the patient needs a referral from his or her primary care provider to see any specialist; if a patient goes out-of-network without the HMO's approval, the patient must pay out-of-pocket

HMO (health maintenance organization)   patient who uses a health maintenance organization (HMO) pays a fixed yearly fee, and must choose among an approved network of health care providers and hospitals; the patient needs a referral from his or her primary care provider to see any specialist; if the patient goes out-of-network without the HMO's approval, the patient must pay out-of-pocket

Help menu   allows the user to access help

HIPA (Health Insurance Portability and Accountability Act)   the first federal legislation dealing with the privacy of medical information

Hourglass   basic mouse pointer shape; the mouse pointer is an hourglass when the computer is processing a command

Human Genome Project   government-financed project that seeks to understand the genetic makeup of a human being; part of the Human Genome Project attempts to gain an understanding of the genetic bases of diseases

I-beam   basic mouse pointer shape; the mouse pointer is an I-beam when editing data

ICD-9-CM International Classification of Diseases   provides 3-, 4-, or 5-digit codes for more than 1000 diseases; the ICD is the *International Classification of Diseases*, 9th ed.

Icon   a little picture representing programs, commands, or hardware

ILIAD   simulation program that teaches clinical problem-solving skills

Impact printer   a printer that prints by having a print head strike an inked ribbon; a dot-matrix printer is an example of an impact printer

Indemnity plan   fee-for-service insurance plan; patient is never restricted to a network of providers and needs no referrals for specialists; after fulfilling a deductible (a certain amount the patient is required to pay each year before the insurance begins paying), every visit to a doctor is paid for by the insurance company

Information   facts in a form useful to human beings

Ink-jet printer   nonimpact printer; forms characters and graphics by spraying dots of ink on paper

Input device   a device that gets data into a computer; input devices include keyboards and direct-entry devices (pointing devices, scanning devices)

Insertion point   cursor; indicates where the next character, number, or symbol will appear

Insurance aging report   lists claims filed by age

Insurance analysis report   report that lists each insurance carrier that has been billed, amounts and percentages of claims, charges, and payments

Insurance carrier   the company that insures a patient

Internet   a network of networks linking computers and users worldwide

Key field   the field in a table that uniquely identifies each record

Keyboard   an input device

Kilobyte (K, Kb)   about 1,000 bytes

Kurzweil scanner   input device that scans printed text and reads it aloud; an adaptive device

Labels report   a report in mailing labels format

Laser printers   laser printers produce the best output, but are the most expensive; the technology used by laser printers is similar to that used by Xerox machines

Ledger   report that shows activity for each account

Line-of-sight systems   input systems whereby you look at a character for a certain number of seconds and it appears on the screen

List box   element in a dialog box that allows the user to make a choice from a list

Lists menu   contains options that allow the user to enter and edit patient, case, and procedure payment information, adjustment codes, diagnosis, insurance and billing codes, and information on providers and referring providers

Magnetic disk   Secondary storage device that saves information as magnetized or nonmagnetized spots

Magnetic ink character recognition (MICR)   An input (scanning) device used by the banking industry to read the numbers (in magnetic ink) at the bottom of checks

Magnetic resonance imaging (MRI)   imaging device that bounces radio waves off the human body and measures the response; the numbers generated are turned into pictures by the computer; MRI can image soft tissue, unlike a traditional X ray

Magnetic stripe   the magnetic stripe on the back of your credit card contains a little information that can be input to a computer (POS terminal)

Magnetic tape   a sequential access secondary storage medium

Mainframe   a multiuser, fast, and powerful computer; tends to perform input/output intensive tasks such as generating a payroll or insurance claims

Managed care   with managed care, it is the insurance carrier that determines what treatment is necessary and pays for it; in managed care, patients pay a fixed yearly fee; the insurance company pays the participating provider

Maximize button   at the top right-hand corner of the window; clicking on the maximize button causes the window to expand to fill the screen and the maximize button to become a restore button

Medicaid   jointly funded, federal-state health insurance for certain low-income and needy people. Including children, the aged, blind, and/or disabled, and people who are eligible to receive federally assisted income maintenance payments. Medicaid resembles managed care, in that the patient is restricted to a network of providers, must get a preauthorization for procedures, and needs referrals to any specialist

Medical informatics   the use of computer technology in health care and its delivery

Medicare   government-funded health insurance for the elderly and disabled people with chronic renal disorders; Medicare allows patients to choose their physicians; referrals are not needed.

MediSoft   program that helps to computerize a medical office; performs administrative tasks: scheduling, and financial tasks such as billing, submitting claims to insurance companies; stores patient, provider, and transaction data; structure based on a relational database

MediSoft date   the date used by the MediSoft administrator; it may not be today's date

MediSoft sidebar   provides shortcuts to accounting functions, patient and office management tasks and daily reports

MediSoft toolbar (speedbar)   gives the user quick access to common functions

MEDLARS a group of health-related databases maintained by the federal government and free to the public

MEDLINE most comprehensive of the MEDLARS databases

Megabyte (M, Mb) about one million bytes

Megahertz one million clock cycles; clock speed is measured in megahertz; clock speed helps determine the speed of the computer

Memory internal storage, includes RAM, ROM, and cache. ROM is permanent, containing start-up instructions; RAM is temporary, holding the work you are doing and the program you are using, and parts of the operating system; cache holds the next instruction and piece of data you will need

Menu a list of choices

Menu bar below the title bar of a window; menu bar contains the names of menus (file, edit, view, etc.); to access the commands, click on the menu title

Microcomputer or PC is a single-user environment powerful enough for a single user to write papers, even books, do math with spreadsheets, create databases, and presentations—most are connected to the Internet multiplying the power of the PC

Minimize button in the upper right-hand corner of any window; clicking on it causes the window to shrink to the size of a button on the taskbar; the program remains running

Monitor an output device; produces soft copy

Motherboard the main circuit board of the computer

Mouse input device; pointing device

Networking connecting computers to each other

Nonimpact printers form letters by spraying dots of ink on paper; ink-jet printers produce excellent quality text and graphics in black and white and color at a low cost

Office hours MediSoft's appointment scheduler

Operating system (OS) a group of programs that manages the resources of the computer. It controls the hardware, manages basic input and output operations, keeps track of your files saved on disk and in memory, and directs communication between the CPU and other pieces of hardware. It coordinates how other programs work with the hardware and with each other. Operating systems also provide the user interface, that is, the way the user communicates with the computer. For example, Windows provides a graphical user interface.

Optical card optical card is a small portable storage medium that stores data as pits and lands and holds about 2,000 pages of data

Optical disk optical disks are used as secondary storage media; store data as pits and lands burnt into a plastic disk by a laser

Optical character recognition (OCR) input device that reads printed characters

Optical mark recognition (OMR) an input device that can sense a mark by a number 2 pencil on a Scantron sheet

Option button round button in a dialog box; one choice must be made from a set of option buttons

Output device an output device (monitor, printer) takes the zeros and ones that the computer processes and produces information useful to human beings

Pack data compresses data

Password words—strings of letters and numbers—that are given to authorized people so that they can use a computer or network; attempt to protect privacy

Patient aging report   report that lists the patient with the amounts owed to the practice by age

Patient day sheet   lists the day's patients, chart numbers, and transactions; used for daily reconciliation

Patient face sheet   a report listing patient information

Patient ledger   report that displays the status of each patient's account, past activity, and billing history

Patient list   a list of patients and patient information sorted by default in chart number order

Patient recall list   lists patients, their phone numbers, and the date of recall

Patient statement   a report that lists a patient's transactions

Payment   an amount received by the health care provider for a service

Payment day sheet   a grouped report organized by providers; each patient is listed under his or her provider; it shows the amounts received from each patient to each provider

Pen-based systems   input systems that recognize handwriting; they are used in some hospitals to enter comments on a patient's chart

Personal computer (PC)   also called a microcomputer; a single-user computer with enough computing power for one person to write papers or even books, use spreadsheet and database management software, and connect to the Internet

Petabyte (P, Pb)   approximately one quadrillion bytes or 1,048,576 gigabytes

PIN number (personal identification number)   identification number given to an authorized user to help guarantee security of information

Plotter   an output device that produces hard copy by moving pens across paper; used for creating architectural drawings and maps

Point   mouse operation that moves the mouse pointer across the screen

Pointing device   a direct-entry input device; pointing devices include a mouse, trackball, touch screen, and various kinds of pen-based input devices

Positron emission tomography (PET) scan   imaging technology in which a patient is injected with radioactive glucose and the rate at which it metabolizes is measured; studies function, including brain function

Practice analysis report   generated on a monthly basis; a summary total of all procedures, charges, and transactions

Preferred provider organizations (PPOs)   preferred provider organizations (PPOs) may require that the provider get authorization before a procedure is performed; patient with PPO insurance can seek care within an approved network of health care providers who have agreed with the insurance company to lower their charges and accept assignment (the amount the insurance company pays). The patient may pay a small copayment.

Primary claim summary   a report showing the insurance status of claims

Primary insurer   the insurance carrier that is billed first

Printer   output device; creates hard copy. The two major categories are impact and nonimpact.

Privacy   the right to control your own information; with the proliferation of computers and networks, this is becoming harder to do

Procedure   includes tests (such as strep cultures) and treatments

Procedure day sheet   a grouped report organized by procedure; patients who underwent a particular procedure such as a blood sugar lab test are listed under that procedure

Processing unit   hardware that manipulates data (comprised of the central processing unit and internal memory)

Processor the brains of the computer, contains ALU, CU, and memory

Program software; line-by-line instructions for a computer

Purge data permanently remove data

Quick balance a quick summary of a patient's balance

Quick ledger a quick summary of a patient's billing and payment status

QWERTY the most widely used computer keyboard; named for the upper-left row of characters

Random access memory (RAM) the temporary, volatile internal workspace, where the user's work, the program the user is using, and parts of the operating system are stored while the computer is in use. RAM is measured in bytes, kilobytes, megabytes, etc.

Read-only memory (ROM) the permanent internal memory that holds start-up instructions; the user cannot change ROM.

Read/write head the part of a disk drive that moves over the spinning disk and that reads data from (makes a copy of the data to put in RAM) and writes data to (takes what is in RAM and puts it on the disk) the diskette

Rebuild index checks the structure of records

Recalculate balances updates balances to reflect newest entries

Recall list a list of patients needing follow-up appointments in a week, month, or a year; Medi-Soft allows the user to create and edit a patient recall list

Record a collection of fields; all the information about one item in a database table

Relational database an organized collection of data in which tables are linked by sharing a common field

Remainder statement after all insurance carriers have paid, a remainder statement shows what the guarantor is responsible for

Repeating appointments the user can instruct the program to display a date that is any number of days, weeks, months, or years from today's date to make an appointment that needs to be periodically repeated

Report designer program in MediSoft that allows the user to design reports

Report designer grid a grid on which the user can design a report structure, entering a report title, column and page headers, and indicating which data fields from the original file(s) are to be included in the detail lines on the report

Reports menu allows the user to access reports or create report structures

Restore button button at the top right-hand corner of the window that allows the user to restore the window to its previous size

Restore data loads backup data onto a computer

Right-click mouse operation that generally opens a shortcut menu

ROM *see* read-only memory

Save put a copy of your work on disk (or another secondary storage medium)

Scanning devices direct-entry input devices, including the optical mark reader, optical character recognition devices, magnetic ink character recognition hardware, Kurzweil scanner, and others

Schedule of benefits a list of those services that the carrier will cover

Scroll bar at the side or bottom of a window, allows the user to move quickly through a document

Secondary insurer the insurance that may pay part of the balance left over after the primary insurer has paid

Secondary storage device   a peripheral device, such as a hard drive, floppy disk drive, zip drive, tape drive or CD drive into which the user inserts a storage medium on which the user can save information permanently

Secondary storage medium   magnetic disk or tape or optical media on which data and information can be saved for long periods of time

Security   security measures attempt to protect computer hardware and software, data and information from being tampered with. Security measures include locking the computer room and distributing keys or swipe cards to authorized personnel. Personnel may be given PIN numbers (personal identification numbers) and passwords. Biometric methods may be used.

Sensor   a device that collects data directly from the environment and sends it to a computer; sensors are used to collect patient information for clinical monitoring

Sequential access storage medium   tape is a sequential access storage medium. To get to the 500th piece of information on tape, you need to fast forward through the first 499.

Shortcut bar   function help line; that contains commonly used function keys

Sidebar   allows the user quick access to accounting functions, patient and office management tasks, and daily reports

Slide box   an element in a dialog box that allows the user to move a pointer to control the speed of, for example, a screen saver

Smart card   card that contains a microprocessor chip and memory. It can do some processing and hold about thirty pages worth of data. Smart cards are used as debit cards.

Soft copy   speech output and the output that appears on a monitor

Software   programs; the line-by-line instructions that tell the hardware what to do; the software that makes a computer such a flexible machine

Special-purpose applications   computer applications in health care that include the use of digital technology in teaching and some aspects of pharmacy

Speech input system   allows you to enter input and commands by speaking to your computer

Speech output system   produces soft copy in the form of speech-like sounds; uses a voice synthesizer program

Speedbar   toolbar; allows the user to access functions quickly

Spin box   an element of a dialog box that allows the user to select a number by clicking on a down arrow or up arrow

Standard toolbar   an element of most windows; contains icons for common operations, such as an open icon, new icon, save and print icons, etc.; allows the user to perform these operations with a click of a mouse

Start button   at the far left-hand corner of the taskbar; allows access to most programs

Status bar   at the bottom of a window; gives context-specific information

Superbill (encounter form)   a list of diagnoses and procedures common to the practice. Superbills for each patient on a day's schedule are printed on that morning or the night before. Information taken from the superbill is utilized in several MediSoft accounting reports.

Supercomputer   largest and most powerful computer; used for processor-intensive tasks, such as weapons research, medical research, weather forecasting, and complex simulations

System clock   a clock that produces a steady beat that is used to synchronize computer operations. Its speed is measured in megahertz; the faster the clock, the faster the computer, all other things being equal

System software   software, including the operating system that controls basic input and output, manages memory and other storage areas, and manages processor time

System unit   hardware; includes the CPU (central processing unit) and internal memory

Tab   an element of a several-page dialog box, allowing access to each page

Table   an organized collection of records

Taskbar   across the bottom of the desktop; contains the start button and a button for every open program; allows the user to move from program to program with a click of the mouse

Telemedicine   the use of telecommunications lines in health care and its delivery

Terabyte (T, Tb)   about one trillion bytes

Text box   an element of a dialog box that allows the user to enter text

Title bar   at the top of the window; contains the window title

Toolbar   displays icons which provide shortcuts to execute commands

Tools menu   gives the user access to a calculator and allows the user to view files

Transactions   charges, payments, and adjustments

TRICARE   federal health benefits program that supplements medical care in the military

Two-headed arrow   mouse pointer shape; the mouse becomes a two-headed arrow for changing the size of a window

User interface   the way the user communicates with the computer, for example, by pointing to an icon and clicking with a mouse

Walkout receipt   the receipt a patient receives after paying at the health care provider's office

Window menu   allows the user to see what windows are open

Window title   across the top of a window in the title bar

Windows   an operating system with a graphical user interface

Windows system date   the date set in Windows; usually today's date

Word processing software   software that allows the user to enter text, edit it, format it, save and retrieve it, and print it

Word size   the number of bits a processor can work with as one unit

Worker's Compensation   a government program that covers job-related illness or injury

World Wide Web   portion of the Internet that is graphical, made up of pages linked to other pages

Index